Unders
Social V
History and

Understanding Social Work

History and Context

John Pierson

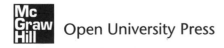 Open University Press

Open University Press
McGraw-Hill Education
McGraw-Hill House
Shoppenhangers Road
Maidenhead
Berkshire
England
SL6 2QL

email: enquiries@openup.co.uk
world wide web: www.openup.co.uk

and Two Penn Plaza, New York, NY 10121-2289, USA

First published 2011

A catalogue record of this book is available from the British Library

ISBN-13: 978-0-335-23795-1 (pb)
ISBN-10: 0-335-23795-9 (pb)
eISBN: 978-0-335-24028-9

Library of Congress Cataloging-in-Publication Data
CIP data applied for

Typeset by Aptara Inc., India
Printed in the UK by Bell & Bain Ltd, Glasgow

Fictitious names of companies, products, people, characters and/or data that may be
used herein (in case studies or in examples) are not intended to represent any real
individual, company, product or event.

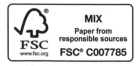

The McGraw·Hill Companies

To Barbara Jones and in memory of Joe Jones
her husband.

Together they looked after a generation of foster children placed with them by Cheshire Social Services. Many children came their way – on long stay or short, in emergency or through well planned placement. Day or night, they were ready to serve.

Theirs is an altruism that we do well to remember and cherish. They are the embodiment of the gift relationship: selfless, dedicated and warmly affectionate. It is upon their actions and attitudes – and of the many like them – that the well-being of looked-after children in Britain depends.

Contents

Acknowledgements   viii

Introduction   x

PART ONE
In the Shadow of the Poor Law   1

1   Forerunners of Social Work   5

2   The Charity Organisation Society   18

**3   The Expanding World of Social Work: Settlements and
       Guilds of Help**   35

4   Social Work between the Wars   50

5   Working with 'Mental Deficiency'   65

6   The Welfare of Children   84

PART TWO
The Road to Modernization   105

**7   Social Work At High Tide: From the Second World War to
       Single Social Services Department**   107

8   Radical Voices, Turbulent Times   127

9   Commissioning, Competences and 'Social Care'   148

10   Social Work with Children and Young People   163

11   From Poor Law to Personalization: Social Work with Adults   186

12   Conclusion: Understanding Social Work History   205

Bibliography   217
Index   235

Acknowledgements

I am grateful to the many who have helped me bring this history together. I would like to thank Chris Hanvey, now head of the Royal College of Paediatricians and Child Health, and Terry Philpot, freelance journalist, for our long-running conversations over many years regarding the nature of social work and its direction of travel. It was and is a privilege to be within their circle. Terry supplied me with many contacts, sources and articles for which I must especially thank him.

I must also thank Martin Thomas, practice educator at Manchester University and valued collaborator, for our regular discussions about the social work scene. He provided me with much of the material on the social work strike in Birmingham in 1978 and has read and commented on a draft of that chapter.

I would particularly like to thank Tom White, former director of Coventry Social Services Department and later chief executive of NCH, who welcomed me into his home for a fascinating discussion of social work from the late 1950s on. Tom kindly sent me his memoirs before they were published and supplied me with the Seebohm Implementation Group's 'Notes for Speakers'.

I would like to thank Craig Cawthorn, former District Manager for Cheshire Social Services, for two lengthy conversations stretching over several hours and for email exchanges on top of that. Craig gave me my first job in social work – as I wrote this volume I could not help but recall with emotion the various high points of my work for Cheshire Social Services in the 1970s and 1980s. For that chance, as well as for the help on this book, I owe him thanks.

I must also thank John Webb, former Director of Adult Services for the Wirral. Our lengthy conversation helped me to situate the development of adult services through the 1990s and the first decade of the twenty-first century.

I am grateful to Margot Webb, former Children's Manager for Cheshire West, for helping me to understand how children's services evolved in the

1990s and early 2000s, as those services negotiated the difficult reefs of crisis and constant reorganization that faced them over the past twenty years.

Anyone who thinks that libraries can safely be cut without significant cultural damage has never written a book. To Marilyn Brookfield at the Bishop Heber High School branch of Cheshire Libraries in Malpas I owe a great deal. Not only did she track down volumes from the dawn of social work in the 1870s onwards, but she would ensure that I returned them all on time. By the time this book appears she will have retired; I am so glad she stayed at the helm until the book was finished.

I would like to thank the anonymous reviewer for the helpful and perceptive comments on an earlier draft of the volume. I would also like to thank Katherine Hartle at Open University Press whose guidance on the book has been greatly appreciated, and Steve Bell who gave me permission to use two of his early cartoons.

Finally, I would like to thank Miriam Sharp Pierson for designing and producing the timelines. She also set up my bibliography for me, saving hours of work, as any author will know.

Introduction

The historical development of social work is an essential but neglected element of our understanding of the profession. The aim here is to correct that, to provide within a single volume an account of the evolution of practice and institutions that led us to where we are today. The volume covers the practical advances, ideas and concepts that practitioners have drawn on over the course of the century and a half of that history. It sets out to restore the long view of social work to our thinking about practice and provision.

History, as Simon Schama has reminded us, is not a placebo, nor 'a stroll down memory lane to escape the headaches of the present'. Rather, history is, by definition, a bone of contention, but it helps us make the distinction between the inessential and the indispensable in our institutions. The alternative is to be held 'in the eternal cage of Now' (Schama 2010).

There are many reasons why the evolution of social work has been neglected. In part it is a result of the focus on 'what works', that is, what works today, not what worked yesterday. Within social work education there is a sense that in a crowded curriculum there is little time to discuss how social work evolved. Organizations are respected and effective only as they build up a reputation for accumulated expertise – but current approaches undermine this at every turn. They learn fast and forget almost as quickly in a hectic 'meetings culture' which damages institutional memory. Beyond this is the latent belief that only the present matters among practitioners, managers and educators alike – that the work undertaken today is in fact superior to that of the past, more enlightened than what has gone before. All therefore that need be done is to improve on the present.

Worshipping the present produces an ever-shrinking window of time, as what is defined as the 'present' becomes ever smaller and what appears to be innovative and noteworthy subject to a brief lifespan: the latest 'innovative projects' last, on average, eighteen months within the organization that gave rise to them, and within two years *have sunk without trace* even within the departments in which they had been located (Pollitt 2008).

This volume then counterposes the awareness of history, of the long-term development of social work to the short-term, constant search for what is 'new'. It shows how the history of social work matters: the importance and persistence of organizational culture, the need for expertise based on accumulated experience, the need to learn systematically from earlier similar events. Social work concerns are cyclical and repeating, and earlier generations worked through their complexity in ways and with experiences that we are foolish to ignore. The job of the critical historian is to consider the evidence, search for patterns and trends over time and discuss plausible interpretations so we can understand what social work is as fully and accurately as possible. Can it be objective? That is unlikely – history is essentially a narrative, and narration requires a point of view. Historical change is contingent and rarely foreordained. Nevertheless the volume aspires to an account that seeks to limit bias, to be transparent in how it renders the narrative and, most importantly, to leave the reader with sufficient materials to shape and produce their own viewpoint. The late US senator Daniel Patrick Moynihan used to say that 'Everyone is entitled to their own views, but they are not entitled to their own facts.' Facts exist – but the selection and organization of those facts will often depend on the viewpoint of the author. History is both a form of truth and a matter of opinion.

Where did social work's major, shaping ideals and ideas on society, power, institutions and human behaviour come from? To discern these is an important endeavour, more than ever needed as the difference between generations of practitioners becomes more pronounced – an older generation, now leaving the scene, that remembers the place of social work within the 'classic welfare state' (and its publicly accepted, even praised, role), and a younger generation that knows only cost centres, the division between commissioners of services and providers of those services in the mixed economy of care and the blurring of public and private service.

A critical history of social work will not resolve the dilemmas facing the profession. What history does provide is a deeper, richer perspective in understanding where and how these dilemmas arose. Readers unfamiliar with this history will encounter profound and energetic practitioners and thinkers who, just like them, were wrestling with difficult and near insoluble problems thrown up by society, who were struggling with issues of war and peace, of social justice, of race and racialized thinking, of stigmatizing disability. They will be astonished also at the range of issues that earlier generations of social work thinkers and doers encountered and deliberated: citizenship, user participation, limits to intrusion into individual privacy, the endless perplexities around youth crime, the relationship between voluntary sector and public sector, how to build collective action out of a service that is in essence based on individuals. They will be heartened by the sheer range and strength of their forebears who, with little prospect of grace or favour, pressed on against the challenges their society faced.

The history of social work is a series of arguments to be debated, not a set of facts to be memorized. Interpreting and understanding those arguments is at the heart of what this volume is trying to do. To meet this purpose it acquaints the reader with the thoughts and practice at the time in order to get her or him thinking about the dilemmas as they appeared and to begin to form their own interpretation. History teaches us about ourselves; it also imparts specific skills: how to ask questions, how to seek out answers and how to think lucidly and purposefully. For professionals it also provides an identity, bearings in a complex present. By asking who we are and how we got here we begin to acquire critical judgement.

The book's plan

The book is based on an accumulation of source materials across a century and a half – books, pamphlets, articles by both prominent and less well known authorities, the minutiae of case notes and other records on how to perform social work. This record has been bolstered by secondary works and wide-ranging interviews with those who have played an important role across many decades in the development of social work services. My own practice experiences, private records and private collection of publications have also played their part.

The development of social work from its beginnings to the present is a vast field – with abundant material that constantly seeks to overflow its banks. I hope the reader will recognize that to render this huge canvas in one volume presents an immense challenge. There is a dilemma in organizing the material – whether to do so in terms of work with user groups or to present it in chronological order. Following the first option the volume could have had single lengthy chapters on children's services, adult services, professional development and so on. Following the second option the chapters would be organized chronologically – origins, the interwar years, the years of the classic welfare state, the challenges of the 1980s and so forth, where the dominant elements of social work in any one period are brought to the fore. Each approach has its strengths. Chapters based on individual services would provide concentrated accounts of those services but would lose the sense of historical development of social work as a whole. Chronological organization, that is following the social work story decade by decade, would provide a readily understood structure but would lead to short summaries of specific fields of practice in any one chapter.

The challenge of a single volume, as far as this author is concerned, is to introduce the reader to the varieties of social work, including its pioneers, whether known or unsung, and at the same time to reflect the big changes in context that affected social work's development from its beginnings to the present. To do this, a mix of both of the above approaches is necessary. Thus the book is divided into two broad parts within which substantive developments of social work as a whole and of particular fields of service are explained and examined. The intention is to give the reader a sense of the broad developments within the evolution of social work and a discussion of the evolution of specific services.

The first part, 'In the Shadow of the Poor Law', covers the period from social work's origins in the nineteenth century through to 1939. The reach of the 1834 Poor Law and its ethos and values, was enormous, affecting all areas of practice in social work's early days; it relinquished its grip only reluctantly during the first half of the twentieth century, and remained a powerful force with which social work had to grapple throughout this entire period. The second part, 'The Road to Modernization', covers the period from 1939 to the present, during which social work became first an adjunct to the welfare state after 1945 and then had to refind its footing in recent decades as provision gave way to market-oriented forces and increased demands and targets from central government.

Chapter 1 looks at the precursors of social work in the various schemes for district-based organization of home visiting the poor. Chapter 2 then examines the rise of the Charity Organisation Society (COS) in the latter part of the nineteenth century; the COS was the first organization that we can directly trace social work's lineage back to, and for several decades was the standard bearer of generic casework. Chapter 3 discusses the settlement house movement and other critics of the COS approach. Chapter 4 looks at social work between the world wars, that is, from 1919 to 1939. It examines the consolidation of social work 'method' around casework in the 1920s and how this effort to develop a credible expertise prompted attempts to become a fully fledged profession.

The next two chapters cover the development of specific services for what, in effect, were the two major 'client' or user groups of the time: 'mental defectives' – people with learning disabilities – and impoverished families. Chapter 5 looks at the evolution of practice concerning people with learning disability and mental health problems. In a sense this was the first specialist social work service to emerge out of the generic approach of its origins. It is difficult for us now to understand how all-encompassing the notion of 'mental defective' was in the first half of the twentieth century, and this chapter recounts the extraordinary unease in government and within public opinion makers and social work itself that surrounded learning disability, particularly within working-class families. Chapter 6 looks at the risks facing children in the late nineteenth and the first half of the twentieth century and how social work organizations, public opinion and statutory authorities gradually moved, at least in part, beyond the Poor Law system in order to respond to these issues. It deals specifically with the issue of 'unmarried mothers' – and children born out of wedlock – and the care and protection of children, including the first steps in developing fostering and adoption.

Part Two, 'The Road to Modernization', follows the development of social work from the Second World War to the threshold of the twenty-first century. It follows the same pattern as Part One, with general chapters in chronological sequence on overall developments in social work. These mark the distance that social work had come and the distance it still had to travel to reach a position where clients were viewed as citizens. Chapter 7 covers the impact of the Second World War on social work, the influence of psychoanalysis and its position within the newly formed welfare state. Chapter 8 examines what is generally regard as the high tide of social work: the establishment of generic social services departments under local authority control as recommended by the Seebohm Committee in 1968. Chapter 9 considers the ferment and dissent of the 1970s with the emergence of radical social work on the one hand and the heightened hostility to social work from sections of the media and political arena, on the other. Chapter 10 considers the developments of services for children and families, from the creation of the children's departments in 1948 and their amalgamation into social services departments in the 1970s to the impact of recurrent child abuse scandals on the service and the reforms initiated by the Children Acts 1989 and 2004. Chapter 11 covers the same span of time with regard to adult services. These services are now distinct in their work with particular user groups – older people, those with mental health problems, and people with learning and physical disability.

In general the volume encourages the reader to reach their own interpretation throughout the century and a half of social work history. But, as I say above, history is about interpreting arguments and viewpoints, and Chapter 12 concludes the volume by offering different ways of interpreting that history and draws out some of the prominent themes in social work's development.

Part One
In the Shadow of the Poor Law

SOCIAL WORK TIMELINE
1819-1939

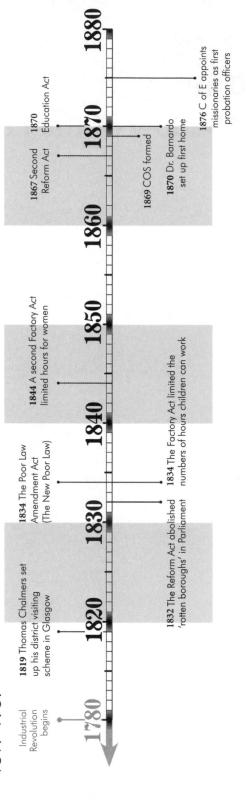

1819 Thomas Chalmers set up his district visiting scheme in Glasgow

Industrial Revolution begins

1832 The Reform Act abolished 'rotten boroughs' in Parliament

1834 The Poor Law Amendment Act (The New Poor Law)

1834 The Factory Act limited the numbers of hours children can work

1844 A second Factory Act limited hours for women

1867 Second Reform Act

1870 Education Act

1869 COS formed

1870 Dr. Barnardo set up first home

1876 C of E appoints missionaries as first probation officers

1780   1820   1830   1840   1850   1860   1870   1880

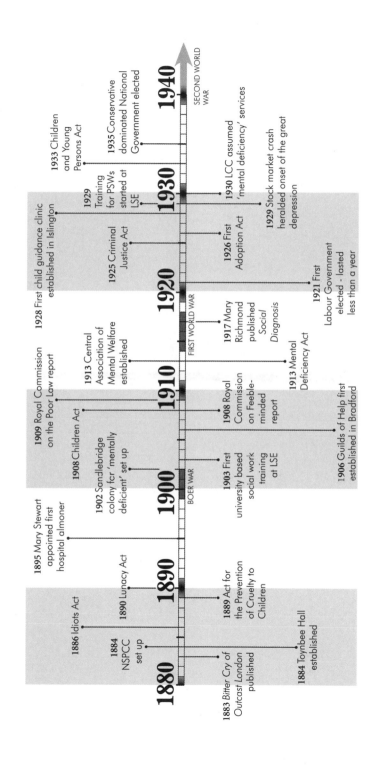

1880

1883 Bitter Cry of Outcast London published

1884 NSPCC set up

1884 Toynbee Hall established

1886 Idiots Act

1890 Lunacy Act

1889 Act for the Prevention of Cruelty to Children

1890

1895 Mary Stewart appointed first hospital almoner

1900

BOER WAR

1902 Sandlebridge colony for 'mentally deficient' set up

1903 First university based social work training at LSE

1906 Guilds of Help first established in Bradford

1908 Children Act

1909 Royal Commission on the Poor Law report

1910

1913 Central Association of Mental Welfare established

1908 Royal Commission on Feeble-minded report

1913 Mental Deficiency Act

FIRST WORLD WAR

1917 Mary Richmond published *Social Diagnosis*

1920

1928 First child guidance clinic established in Islington

1925 Criminal Justice Act

1921 First Labour Government elected - lasted less than a year

1926 First Adoption Act

1929 Training for PSWs started at LSE

1930

1933 Children and Young Persons Act

1935 Conservative dominated National Government elected

1930 LCC assumed 'mental deficiency' services

1929 Stock market crash heralded onset of the great depression

1940

SECOND WORLD WAR

1 Forerunners of Social Work

This chapter discusses the beginnings of social work by looking at how the industrial revolution turned British society upside down within the space of a few decades in the early nineteenth century and how the social problems that emerged from that revolution were the seedbed for social work itself. It explores:

- the framework of values and institutions that the New Poor Law established in the 1830s to deal with the problems of industrialization;
- how that framework was inextricably linked to the emergence of social work as a distinct form of charity;
- some of social work's charitable precursors and their impact on later developments.

The industrial revolution and its consequences

Britain was the first country to industrialize and the first therefore to have to grapple with the social problems associated with industrialization. The mass migration from countryside to city produced a unique set of challenges that emerged within the space of a single lifetime. From approximately 1780 to 1830 the country went through wrenching upheaval – in society, economics and politics. Family life in urban areas became dominated by mill and factory, by jerry-built housing and poor sanitation while, in rural areas, farm workers' wages were cut. Mechanization and the introduction of steam-powered machinery were drivers of this process, as was the pursuit of profit margins.

In dealing with the many social problems that flowed from this revolution – extensive child labour, poor sanitation, urban epidemics especially cholera – there was no roadmap and no other country's experience to look to. In this respect Britain stood alone. The staggering growth in the urban population, and in particular the number of urban poor, provided the seismic centre of a vast social upheaval. In 1801 Manchester had a population of 75,000; by 1841 its population was 235,000. Glasgow, Liverpool and Birmingham had similar growth. Working-class families struggled to gain a foothold in this new economy. Working conditions in factory and mine were harsh and the hours long. Poorly built, back-to-back housing resulted in over-crowding in small cellar rooms or single rooms for large families – in dwellings with little light, and no sewage system or running water.

'The dismal science'

Accompanying this social and economic shock was the rapid growth of a new way of looking at society, and in particular at social problems and how government should, or should not, respond to them. This philosophy (or ide-ology) was broadly called 'laissez-faire' – 'leave it alone' – meaning government should not interfere in the running of the economy. The doctrine spread with lightning speed in the early 1800s throughout the governing, intellectual and economic elites engineering this revolution. And it transformed social policy towards people living in poverty. It had many advocates who, in a cascade of writing from pamphlets to learned tomes, from speeches to parliamentary commissions, promoted the new ideas with a swiftness and zeal that is as-tounding to us even today.

Laissez-faire emphasized that only the marketplace should determine who produces what and at what price and, moreover, that the market should not be subject to any state intervention or state regulation whatsoever. This ap-plied to the labour market, where workers' time, skills and physical effort – their labour power – were bought for wages. For example, the contracts that employers such as coal mine owners, or cotton mill owners, arranged with their employees were regarded purely as a transaction between the individual and the employer and should not in any way be subject of interference from the state. Workers should be free to sell their labour power at the highest rate they could command, and employers should be free to buy that labour at the cheapest price (lowest wage) they could command. Market forces – the mil-lions of negotiations between buyers and sellers, untouched by any kind of regulation – should be free to set the prevailing wage rates.

That markets should be left completely free to operate on their own was not a matter of ideology, said its proponents, but of scientific laws. David Ricardo (1772–1823), a leading economist of the time, thought that wages would inexorably be driven down to near subsistence level as a result of market forces, which was why some commentators at the time referred to political economy as 'the dismal science'. The operation of the labour market, harsh as it could be, was the consequence of natural laws about which nothing could or should be done.

Such was the power of laissez-faire doctrine that the many evident abuses in factories, mills and mines took decades to put right. Some employers, for ex-ample, regarded children as good labourers – they were cheap, they could work long hours, their fingers were nimble and they could fit into spaces that adults could not. Owners of mines and mills found them a huge asset – for example the south Staffordshire pit owners whose coal shafts were particularly narrow – as did parents themselves, such as a widow suddenly left on her own with young male children and no income. It took decades of parliamentary hearings and passionate groups from outside government to pressure Parliament to pass the first Act limiting the number of hours that children could work.

The Factories Acts of 1833 and 1844

The Factories Act 1833 limited the working day for 14–18-year-olds to 12 hours (with an hour lunch break) and limited the working day for 9–13-year-olds to 8 hours and an hour lunch break. It also required employers of children to provide two hours of education – a provision routinely ignored. It outlawed the employment of children aged under 9 in the textile industry.

The Factories Act of 1844 applied the provisions of the 1833 Act to women but *extended* the permitted working day for 9–13-year-olds (and women) to 9 hours.

The 1844 Act also required all accidental deaths to be reported to a surgeon for investigation. Owners were required to wash down workplaces with lime every 14 months.

Thus the picture in the early nineteenth century is of a piece: rapid movement from country to city, poorly built urban housing, poor sanitation and the doctrine of laissez-faire all arrived, historically speaking, at about the same time and utterly transformed the large urban centres of manufacturing and trade such as Liverpool, Manchester, Sheffield and Birmingham. While we use the phrase 'industrial revolution' to describe the process in a far away time, for those living through it, it was an unprecedented upheaval which took place well within the lifetime of individuals.

The Poor Law Amendment Act 1834 – the 'New Poor Law'

At the outset of the industrial revolution the relief of poverty was based wholly on the individual parish and had been so since the passage of the 1601 Elizabethan Poor Law. Under this statute, people who were completely destitute and facing starvation applied to their own parish for relief, which was provided in kind or in cash by local rate – tax – payers. This arrangement reflected a reasonably settled social world, based on hierarchy and traditional forms of authority maintained in localities by the Church of England and by local justices of the peace drawn from the gentry to enforce the law. At the top sat the royal court and the great aristocratic houses; at the bottom was the great percentage of the population most of which had never left their parish (Hobsbawm 1988).

The industrial revolution upended this small-scale, essentially face-to-face welfare system. While it generated untold wealth for the entrepreneurs and businessmen who consolidated the technology around steam-powered cotton mills or factory-scale textile production, it also generated poverty on an epic scale – and the challenge of paying for the extensive poor relief on the basis of the old system, especially in the urban districts, that came on the back of the revolution was too great. There were also ideological reasons behind the campaign for a new Poor Law – the belief that the old welfare system had been too accommodating of the able-bodied poor, providing supplements to wages in the form of bread and inappropriate cash handouts to those who did not deserve them.

Following the report from the Royal Commission into the Operation of the Poor Laws, Parliament undertook root and branch reform that completely transformed the nature of poor relief across Britain. The Act, passed in 1834 – technically the Poor Law Amendment Act (that is, amending the earlier Elizabethan statute) – introduced quite different arrangements for poor relief based on the following principles:

1. Any relief of destitute people should be set at a level *below* the lowest level of wages earned by able-bodied labourers; this was the principle of 'less eligibility', that is, the life of any one receiving poor relief should be less satisfactory than that of the lowest paid labourer. Its aim was to create a sense of social stigma, the stigma of 'pauperism': in a society where the great percentage of people were poor, only 'paupers' – those so destitute that they were compelled to go into the workhouse – became objects of shame in their own eyes and the eyes of others. In this the framers of the Act succeeded.

2. The new system should have a strong element of deterrence for those individuals thinking of applying for poor relief, ensuring that anyone would have to be living at a subsistence level to do so. Deterrence came in the form of the workhouse. To receive poor relief, people would have to enter the workhouse where the regime was spartan. Diet was based on bread and gruel, sleeping quarters were communal and daytime occupied by hard labour – for women, including older women, picking old rope hemp (oakum), whereas male inmates broke stones.

3. The old parish basis for relief would be abolished and parishes grouped together in larger Poor Law Unions overseen by a board of guardians who in turn were regulated by the Poor Law Commission based in London.

In practice there were further deterrents from seeking relief under the Act. In particular, children were separated from their mothers, and older married couples from one another. But not all workhouse regimes were as hard as the law intended. Some Poor Law Unions offered assistance outside the workhouse ('outdoor relief'); others, with time, acknowledged that different groups of paupers had different needs and so provided schools for children and infirmaries for the sick.

In Scotland the system was different where there was a substantial tradition of outdoor relief. From 1845 the authorities were encouraged to form 'combinations' of parishes as in England that could also build workhouses if they so wished. But the option of out relief was explicit and continued to be the preferred option of Scottish poor law authorities. The introduction of Poor Law principles in Ireland in the 1840s took the opposite path – unlike England, Wales and Scotland outdoor relief was explicitly forbidden; the poor law authorities there administered the principles of 1834 with a ruthless consistency that contributed significantly to the great famine that over took the country in the mid 1840s resulting in the deaths of approximately one million people – and the emigration (largely to the US) of another million resulting in an overall loss of population estimated between 20 and 25 per cent.

Forerunners of social work

Alongside the industrial revolution a moral revolution, largely based on the rising middle class and forms of evangelical Christianity, erupted in Britain in the same decades from 1780 onwards. The range of activities that flowed from disparate movements had an astonishing sweep: prison reform, abolition of the slave trade, the temperance movement, suppression of vice and prostitution, reform of mental health institutions, campaigns against cruelty to animals, among others. Powerful voluntary organizations emerged in its wake: the Society for Prevention of Cruelty to Animals, Prison Discipline Society, Anti-Slavery Society, the Vice Society, and many others.

In the main, the work of these societies was created, developed and furthered by an expanding middle class motivated by a renewed sense of personal responsibility and a determination to tackle the social problems that came in the wake of industrialization.

The activists came from across professional, religious, judicial ranks – bankers, magistrates, industrialists, entrepreneurs, clergymen, publicists, lawyers. Today we may understand the word 'evangelical' differently – then it was used to capture this broad, energetic, Protestant-based reform movement. There were many strands within it – Anglican, Quaker, Unitarian, Methodist – with different visions of society. Some groups inclined towards a more hierarchical and paternalistic view of society, others were more plural and democratic; some were sectarian, others ecumenical in outlook. But they held in common the propriety of family life and, above all, the necessity of engaging in voluntary activity to further social reform.

In terms of poor relief, the reform movement shared the goals of the Poor Law reform. Its advocates thought that poverty arose through weakness of individual moral character and lack of responsibility. They wanted to see pauperism extinguished, but their values were different from the cold arguments of economic efficiency put forward by the likes of Ricardo and other protagonists of pure laissez-faire. They regarded the operation of the marketplace as a test of moral character, and their efforts were focused accordingly on the need to assess individual character by whether or not individual persons applying for poor relief had been responsible for their own poverty. Nor could the process of discriminating individual character be reduced to an impersonal test such as the 'less eligibility' requirement in the New Poor Law: it could only be determined through personal contact.

Social work emerged from this movement, but there are difficulties in attempting to pinpoint any one specific precedent. Lady Derby's Benevolent Society of Annual Sale of Ornamental and Fancy Works was begun in 1829 – when her Ladyship and other respectable women of Liverpool became shopkeepers for the day to sell articles to purchasers, with the money raised going to a range of local charities (Simey 1951: 28). In no stretch could that be called social work. But the work of the District Provident Society in Liverpool probably could be. It acknowledged the difficulty of preaching Christianity to men and women 'who have no comforts and seemingly no desire for any, who live with, and like pigs in miserable, wet, unwholesome cellars, hot beds of disease without any provisions for the next meal' (Simey 1951: 30), and gets closer to something we might recognize as social work because it introduced personal contact between the women visitors and the individual poor families.

District Provident Society in Liverpool

The District Provident Society drew on 200 helpers, organized into 21 district committees. The Society gave sixpence to impoverished individuals for every ten shillings they saved, along with advice on conduct and morals. The Society was also preoccupied with the moral shortcomings of the poor – and tended in time to become a society for the suppression of vice rather than for the promotion of virtue. 'A word spoken in season every week by a rich person to a poor person, will do more to reclaim him from reckless improvidence and low debauchery than any other human expedient that I know', said the Society's agent in 1829 (quoted in Simey 1951: 30).

Through the first half of the nineteenth century a hardening attitude towards the poor – with calls for tougher, more discriminating forms of charity – emerged in tandem with the advent of the 'New Poor Law'. Through the middle decades of the nineteenth century, poverty continued to be viewed by the middle-class supporters of voluntary associations as a moral condition, that is, a consequence of irresponsibility and lack of foresight in the individual concerned. How else to explain the fact of extensive poverty in the midst of Victorian plenty? In the wake of this perspective came numerous efforts, often faith based, to rouse the poor from their bad choices and culture of poverty. Social work began to emerge as urban missions developed *relationships* with individuals, aiming to put themselves in 'close sympathy' with the wants and feelings of the poor while at the same time acting as moral adviser and friend to promote responsible behaviour.

The Reverend John Johns (1801–1847)

In his short life Johns demonstrated the passion of a social reformer, envisaging remedies and social responses that were well ahead of his time. He was not so bothered by his modest success but that he could show that some achievement was possible. In 1836 he was invited from Dorset to lead the Domestic Mission work for the Unitarians in Liverpool.

> His days were largely spent in visiting the homes of his poor neighbours whenever opportunity offered, of which visits he kept careful record, quoting them by way of illustration to his Reports. As and when opportunity occurred, small groups were gathered together and simple facilities for such activities as reading provided, on the principle which he evolved from his own experience, that 'the most precious good that can be done for the poor is that which you can induce them to do for themselves'.
>
> (Simey 1951: 37)

In the Domestic Mission Report for 1837 Johns wrote:

> I have often found their physical wants so great, as not merely to embitter life, but to antedate its close. I have no hesitation in saying, that an unsuspected amount of human existence must annually be sacrificed, in this and similar towns, *from simple and absolute starvation.* No jury sits on these neglected remains; no horror-stricken neighbourhood is electrified by the rumour, that one has died among them of cold, and nakedness, and hunger. Obscurity clouds the death-bed; and oblivion rests upon the grave.

> But, unknown as it may be to the world at large, the fact is awfully certain – that not a few of our poor, especially of the aged and infirm, die, winter after winter, of no disease but inanition.
>
> (quoted in Simey 1951: 40)
>
> Despite his compassion Johns thought alms should be used only sparingly and in an emergency; the main need was for sympathy and guidance. What distinguished Johns was his profound belief that a common humanity with the poorest individual should be recognized in a society divided heavily by class.

Thomas Chalmers

Thomas Chalmers (1780–1847) is often credited with creating a scheme of family visiting that provided a model for the development of the Charity Organisation Society some fifty years later (see Chapter 2). He was an economist and charismatic preacher who thought deeply about pauperism (which he detested) and about what a harmonious working-class community would look like. In 1819 he persuaded Glasgow town council to establish a new parish called St Johns which he divided into 25 districts. Each district was overseen by a trained deacon with roughly 50 families (approximately 400 persons) under their care. These deacons – all volunteers – were to be friends and advisers to those living within their district. They were to visit each home in their district regularly, and, should a householder be found in extreme poverty they were to proceed, first, to help them find employment and to check on their spending patterns and, second, failing that, to approach relatives and neighbours for small donations if needed. If these means failed, only then would an applicant be supported by parish funds as long as another deacon agreed. The aim was to develop a neighbourhood culture that rejected pauperism and would assist anyone in their locality to avoid its stigma. To this end the parish fund available for relief was kept deliberately low, to forestall deacons becoming overly generous. Contributions came solely through Chalmer's 'Evening Collection', mostly from local residents who attended his evening service – as opposed to his morning service attended by wealthy Glaswegians who flocked to hear him preach. Chalmers also instituted regular meetings of the deacons in which they exchanged information and advice, measured success and took a roll call of incorrigible paupers who proved beyond help (Young and Ashton 1956; Goodlad 2001).

Chalmers' systematic home visiting scheme was not the only aspect of his example that was influential in the coming decades. He thought that the investigation of individual family circumstances could only be ascertained through individual attention and relationship. He wrote:

> It is not enough that you give money, you must give it with judgment. You must give your time and attention. You must descend to the trouble of examination: for instance, will charity corrupt him into slothfulness? What is his particular necessity? Is it the want of health or the want of employment? Is it the pressure of a numerous family? You must go to the poor man's sick-bed. You must lend your hand to the work of assistance. You must examine his accounts. You must try to recover those wages which are detained by the injustice or the rapacity of the master. You must employ your mediation with his superiors, and represent to them the necessities of the situation.
>
> (quoted in Young and Ashton 1956: 78)

Beyond the visitor paying meticulous attention to individual circumstances, Chalmers was also influential in his conception of the relationship between visitor and visited and what it could achieve. Despite the gulf between middle-class visitor and working-class householder, Chalmers thought that through this relationship the moral autonomy of the household would be enhanced and the recipient freed from mere instinctual motivations. In so doing, as Goodlad observed, he helped to invent a modern liberal and middle-class (rather than traditional and aristocratic) version of paternalism (Goodlad 2001: 10).

Chalmers and other evangelicals supported the notion of the free market and laissez-faire but with a different emphasis from mainstream political economy. They saw the market system as 'retributive and purgative employing competition as a means of education rather than [economic] growth' (Hilton 1988: 68). They believed fiercely that the health of the economy and of the political system depended on observation of a moral code, one that was emphatically Christian. In this context the free market was an impersonal agent of moral law – it allocated resources but it also rewarded virtue and punished vice. It was government's task to remove all constraints on the market so that morality should prevail (Stedman Jones 2004: 178).

Discussion point   Dr Thomas Chalmers

Chalmers was the nineteenth-century equivalent of the Renaissance man, a polymath and one of the central figures of the Scottish Enlightenment of the late eighteenth and early nineteenth centuries. He was a trained mathematician, an economist and an ordained minister in the Church of Scotland. He was also a man of immense energy which he applied in a number of fields of engagement, whether in devising his system of poor relief in Glasgow or as charismatic preacher.

In a letter regarding how volunteers should approach the poor he wrote:

> Be kind and courteous to the people, while firm in your investigations about them; and in proportion to the care with which you investigate will be the rarity of the applications that are made to you .... If drunkenness be a habit with the applicants, this in itself is an evidence of means, and the most firm discouragement should be put upon every application in these circumstances. Many applications will end in your refusal of them in the first instance; because till they have had experience of your vigilance, the most undeserving are apt to obtrude themselves; but even with them shew good-will, maintain calmness, take every way of promoting the interest of their families and gain, if possible their confidence and regard by your friendly advice and the cordial interest you take in all that belong to them.
>
> (quoted in Young and Ashton 1956: 72)

Chalmers stunned his supporters in Glasgow when, after just three years of overseeing his scheme of poor relief, he resigned his living in 1823 to take up a post at Edinburgh University – his scheme was eventually wound up in 1837. He cited exhaustion and illness as the reasons for having to leave so soon. His scheme was not widely appreciated in Glasgow and he was the butt of attacks in the Glasgow press. There may have been other reasons for his abrupt departure, however. Historians have challenged the authenticity of his financial accounts. From her researches, Furgol (1987) maintained that he refused to consider that he might be mistaken, which led him to dismissing any evidence that pointed to his scheme not working. She judged that his experiment in poor relief failed unequivocally and that his ideal small community never actually materialized.

After reading this section on Chalmers do you think his legacy is essentially positive or negative, just or unjust, socially fair or socially divisive? Draw up a list of what you regard as positive and negative in his proposals.

As the 'laws' of political economy became dominant, there was an accompanying drive against public waste, and anxiety over how indiscriminate charity undermined individual independence and responsibility. This posed a dilemma for those organizations that sought to relieve poverty that could be summed up as the struggle between 'heart and head'. The emerging poor relief organizations accepted the principles of what they regarded as natural science but at the same time wanted to signal that it was both the duty of the upper middle class and the Christian thing to do to relieve poverty. Thus charity organizations consciously played a mediating role between the impersonal operation of the labour market (and later the bureaucratic operation of the New Poor Law) and the difficult circumstances that individuals faced when thrown into poverty – giving 'the poor time to adjust and a reason for not losing faith in the benevolent intention of the propertied' (Roberts 2004: 137). They had to wrestle with the fine line between wanting to underpin the discipline of the labour market and yet supporting the needy – ultimately this meant some sort of categorizing of the poor. It is important to remember that in the early nineteenth century nearly everyone was poor. Creating different categories of those in poverty, distinguishing for example between the indolent able-bodied male and the hard-working head of household who had lost his trade through injury, was a crucial step for those wanting to assist in some way. Thus, long before the Charity Organisation Society was formed (see Chapter 2), the notion of the 'deserving' and 'undeserving' poor was well established in charitable practice.

The Mendicity Society grappled with exactly these issues. The Society was formed in 1818 to reduce begging on the streets of London (and eventually other cities). Its practice was to hand out tickets to beggars that they would then submit in exchange for food and night shelter. The organization's logic was that only those who were truly pressed would accept the ticket; beggars that were only interested in a quick cash handout would not. But the Society soon confronted several dilemmas that would echo throughout the nineteenth century. How do you establish the willingness to work when there is no work available? Which is more truly charitable: to provide charity indiscriminately or to use charity as a way of encouraging responsibility, thrift and independence? What about the children of beggars? What about the children who *were* beggars? In the end, by the 1820s the Society moved to professionalize its staff, introduced a standardized test for willingness to work that prefigured the New Poor Law and categorized its applicants as to whether they were deserving or undeserving (Roberts 1991).

Upsurge in charitable activity through voluntary associations

The middle decades of the nineteenth century saw an outpouring of voluntary association activity as the associations grappled with a new social phenomenon: mass urban poverty which threatened to overwhelm the workhouse-based system of poor relief whether charitable or state provided. The sheer number of voluntary associations seeking to instil the principles of moral conduct at the same time as finding ways to relieve the most destitute casualties of the industrial revolution has to be borne in mind. City missions and provident societies proliferated, as did night asylums and soup kitchens for the homeless and societies for repressing mendicity or begging. There were many visiting societies created in Chalmers' wake, with the Church of England, Congregationalists and Methodists all creating organizations that combined visiting poor households with enquiry into their material circumstances along with questions to do with religious affiliation and whether or not the family possessed a Bible.

There are three important points arising from this wave of voluntary organizations. First, the organizations were overwhelmingly local – with exceptions, they were not national or regional. Occasionally they would develop a London-wide association – as with the Metropolitan Visiting and Relief Association formed in 1846 – but on the whole the voluntary effort had the strengths and weaknesses of being local in operation. Yes, they were local and embedded within their communities, but volunteers and funding were often in short supply and the actual reach of their work was frequently limited. Second, they were often in competition with each other in localities competing for voluntary effort and resources. Sectarian antagonisms played their part also, as when faith-based agencies tied charitable giving to their recipients' attending a particular church – and then becoming progressively more generous in their levels of poor relief in order to attract more followers. As societies of all description proliferated, the discipline around the principles for providing monetary relief became more and more diverse. Training was non-existent, and, in the view of those critics of this approach who later formed the Charity Organisation Society, this multiplicity of benevolent activity had strayed too far from Poor Law principles.

By the end of the 1860s, forces were amassing that wanted a return to the principles of 1834. The Poor Law Board (which had replaced the Poor Law Commission in 1847) saw what it regarded as a dangerous trend, particularly in London where 'outdoor relief' – that is, poor relief provided outside the workhouse – had grown substantially as metropolitan Poor Law guardians responded to rising unemployment. This marked the start of an extensive crusade against outdoor relief in which 'lazy' able-bodied males were presumed to be taking advantage of the system. As in so many similar campaigns, those alleged to be taking advantage of the system – the feckless and work-shy able-bodied – on closer inspection were orphans, widows, disabled or the very old. The Poor Law Board issued a call for greater coordination and pressed the newly formed Charity Organisation Society into taking on the task of coordinating both relief under the Poor Law and charitable giving with a brief to cut it drastically.

When the Local Government Board in turn replaced the Poor Law Board in 1871, the campaign accelerated and outdoor relief was cut substantially. Overall the numbers of people on outdoor relief fell from 874,000 in 1871 to 567,000 in 1877. The number of able-bodied men receiving outdoor relief – at whom the crusade was ostensibly aimed – was always a small percentage of those receiving aid but became even smaller, falling from 30,000 (3.4 per cent of all recipients) to 13,000 in the same six years (Humphreys 1995: 31). Certain Poor Law Unions were more zealous than others in pursuing the Local Government Board objectives. Brixworth guardians in Northhamptonshire, for example, saw it as their responsibility to teach the working-class families about their responsibilities towards their poor relations and mounted campaigns for contributions from the relatives of those seeking poor relief. They also abolished outdoor relief for women, including widows with children. This policy necessitated taking a widow's (or unmarried mother's) children into the workhouse – leaving one child behind 'lest the mother would forget her dual role'. This they justified on the basis that 'the woman is set free for work' and the children 'better fed and better disciplined . . . and better taught' (Humphreys 1995: 33).

It was within this context that the Charity Organisation Society, the first organization to which social work today can trace a direct lineage, was called into being and given the task of coordinating both voluntary associational charity and the state provision under the Poor Law.

Summary

- Rapid industrialization led to population surges in urban areas such as Manchester and Liverpool.
- This presented Britain with a range of problems, arising out of a large urban working class on low wages and living in poorly constructed housing, that no other country had previously experienced.
- The New Poor Law of 1834 aimed to create a deterrent to those who would not work for a living; it established a chain of workhouses the regimes of which were deliberately harsh so that only those facing utter destitution would choose to enter.
- A number of district visiting schemes were established in major cities – such as Glasgow, Liverpool and London. Such schemes were designed to provide volunteers who would visit the very poor in their homes to offer advice and support in an effort to get them to live a more industrious and responsible life.

Suggested reading

Roberts, M. J. D. (2004). *Making English Morals: Voluntary Association and Moral Reform in England 1787–1886*. Cambridge: Cambridge University Press.

Young, A. F. and E. T. Ashton (1956). *British Social Work in the Nineteenth Century*. London: Routledge & Kegan Paul.

2   The Charity Organisation Society

This chapter covers the founding of the Charity Organisation Society (COS) and discusses its significance for the development of social work. The COS marks the beginning of what is recognizably social work in the sense that there is a clear line of descent between it and later social work organizations. The chapter discusses:

- the organization and principles of the COS and how it responded to a range of applicants for poor relief;
- the leading thinkers of the COS who were the first to formalize case work as a method;
- the work of hospital almoners – the first medical social workers – as an offshoot of the COS.

Charity Organisation Society: foundation and first decades

By the 1860s significant changes in society and economy had taken place. This was the 'age of equipoise', of balance, with the sense that the rawness of industrial revolution had been tamed, at least in the perception of moral reformers and political elites. Society, particularly in urban areas, was regarded as more in harmony with itself. It was a period of greater affluence, some of which had reached sectors of the skilled working class, the so-called aristocracy of labour. The political upheavals of the 1840s, in which the Chartist agitation for universal suffrage and annually elected parliaments had appeared as dangerously revolutionary, had given way to an increased willingness to give at least some sectors of the working class the right to vote. In 1867 a Conservative government led by Benjamin Disraeli did just that, giving a small section of the urban working class the right to vote in the Reform Act of 1867. It is probably right to conclude, as historians generally have, that the market-based society, underpinned by modest democratic expansion at home and empire abroad, had developed stability and a significant level of popular support (Hoppen 1998).

Yet precisely because of this sense of new-found stability, anxieties about working-class behaviour and its vulnerability to loss of self-control only grew larger in the minds of moral reformers and those administering the Poor Law. Indeed, the rising, but selective level of prosperity and the widening of the franchise demanded that the moral virtues of thrift, individual responsibility and temperate behaviour were even more important. William Ewart Gladstone, leader of the Liberal Party and several times prime minister, explicitly supported extending the franchise only to those who morally qualified, namely those who showed a character of 'self-command, self control, respect for order, patience under suffering, confidence in the law, regard for superiors' (Hoppen 1998: 245).

This was the context in which the Charity Organisation Society was born. While the COS had its precursors in the provident societies and work of Thomas Chalmers, there were specific concerns in the late 1860s regarding the sudden rise in the number of paupers claiming poor relief (in the wake of the recession of 1866) and the link to over-generous and ill-disciplined charity that provided the immediate impetus for its founding. A paper presented by a Unitarian minister, Henry Solly, to the Royal Society of Arts in 1868 is generally credited with prompting a number of individuals to come together to form a more rigorous, 'scientific' organization.[1] In a sense this was the trigger for a move that was waiting to happen. Solly's proposal fell on the ready ears of a host of moral reformers, in the main Anglican, and supporters of the strict administration of the Poor Law according to its original principles. Their lengthy experience in London of distress relief through the 1850s and 1860s had renewed the question of dependency of those receiving relief, especially as funds for financing poor relief in east London had been almost exhausted. This objective was also taken up by the president of the Poor Law Board, J. G. Goschen, who issued a lengthy letter, the so-called Goschen Minute, in late 1869, urging coordination between voluntary charity and the Poor Law authorities in order to bring comprehensive discipline to the amount of money being given to paupers, whether from Poor Law guardians or charity.

The Society for the Organisation of Charitable Relief and Repressing Mendicity – soon to change its name to the Charity Organisation Society – was formed in that same year, 1869, with the aim to rationalize and coordinate charitable giving, first in London and then in the other large cities. Prominent representatives from the aristocracy, Parliament, banking, the professions and public intellectuals dominated its national council. Queen Victoria became patron in 1874. Twenty-four vice-presidents were added in the early 1870s, providing another cohort of well known figures, including the influential critic John Ruskin and J. G. Goschen, to buttress the Society's work.

The Society moved swiftly to establish district committees, first in London and then in towns and cities such as Birkenhead, Birmingham,

Brighton, Liverpool, Oxford and Manchester. London remained the epicentre of the work. The district committees there remained the more disciplined in following COS principles and provided the base for its leading public intellectuals who wrote extensively advocating for and publicizing the work of the COS. The provincial societies were more diverse, and while they professed commitment to the principles of the Society they were less constrained in their application by the rules announced by London (Humphreys 1995).

The founders of the COS sought a return to the rigour of the 1834 Poor Law by eliminating as far as possible outdoor relief of the poor. From the first, the COS stressed that dependence on relief, whether public or private, must inevitably weaken individual self-reliance and sense of responsibility. It recognized that the sheer number of competing charitable organizations aiming to relieve poverty meant that charitable giving to the poor was lavish and took no account of how indiscriminate charity undermined thrift, responsibility and hard work. The original task of the COS, then, was not to provide charitable relief itself but to coordinate charitable efforts of organizations already in the field and to refer deserving applicants to the appropriate agency where they would find the assistance they needed. It operated, however, under the presumption that most of those seeking relief were attempting to escape their responsibilities, in which case providing relief of any kind would only further encourage this. In what its own historians later described as the 'hard and dry years' – the first decade of its existence, the 1870s – the COS endeavoured to fulfil this mission to the letter (Bosanquet 1901).

The Society was founded at the crest of the crusade against outdoor relief and was the chief representation of it. Some earlier histories of social work have treated the COS as pioneers of social work (which it was), but play down the values and social objectives which it sought to promote. The COS founders, publicists and salaried agents were in close alliance and shared with the Local Government Board and the Poor Law Board the determination to prune outdoor relief as drastically as it could. Its methods were designed to investigate rigorously those who claimed outdoor relief. Any outdoor support it would recommend for families or individuals would be set at levels that encouraged self-sufficiency. Beyond this the Society also assumed that people of a higher social and financial status were naturally also morally, spiritually and intellectually superior. By receiving poor relief *in* the workhouse, recipients would also be submitting to a regime of moral correction.

The COS emphasis on 'character'

Very quickly the COS realized it could confine itself to coordinating charities in a given urban area but had to lead by example in providing poor relief itself. For COS family visitors, the nature of a person's character was the most important element to assess in a family's situation. Helen Bosanquet, a leading thinker of the Society, emphasized how individual character can make one family rich and another poor:

> There is no fact more constantly and impressively borne in upon the minds of those who have seen many people in their home life, that one and the same income will mean comfort in one home and squalor in another. In the one house we find cleanliness and neatness, healthy children and clean faces, a bright hearth and pictures on the wall.... Next door, where possibly more money is actually earned, there is dirt and discomfort, the remnants of one meal are confused with the next, the children are sickly and unclean, the grate is empty and the coal-bill unpaid.
>
> (Bosanquet 1903: 102)

This notion that individual character was the main ingredient in shaping life chances – more than social class, more than wage inequality – was echoed time and again in COS thinking.

Assessment of character entailed observing behaviours deemed random or impulsive; where identified, they were associated with the 'lower self' that focused on immediate gratification. (To be fair to the COS, belief in the importance of character was widespread in mid-Victorian society and certainly not confined to the COS nor even the middle class but was upheld within the working class where notions of honesty, punctuality and hard work were transmitted through Nonconformist chapels, the temperance movement and working-class Sunday schools.)

That such judgments should take place within the context of the relationship of friendly visiting within the close confines of an impoverished family's home was a source of ambivalence in COS thinking. Its practitioners and district committees who made final decisions on whether to provide some form of charitable relief – or to refer the person to the Poor Law authorities – struggled to balance the possibilities of redemption for the specific individual within what they regarded as a culture of poverty set by those who were lazy, preferred to beg and lead a degraded way of life. This ambivalence emerges particularly in the writings of Charles Stewart Loch and Bernard Bosanquet (Helen's husband), whose devotion to the ideal of the good society and belief in human redemption must always be placed alongside some of the moralizing tendencies of the COS (Bosanquet 1895; Lewis 1995b).

Discussion point   Octavia Hill – For or against

Octavia Hill (1838–1912) was an indisputable pioneer of social work. She helped shape the philosophy and practice of the COS, developed and managed housing units for people on low income, introduced training schemes for her volunteers and, later in life, sat on the Royal Commission on the Poor Law, contributing to the majority report in 1909. Some 140 years after she first initiated her housing projects in London her views on poverty and her work are still promoted (Whelan 1998; Prochaska 2006) and still fiercely contested.

Hill was born into a well-off upper middle-class family of Liberal inclination and commitment to public service. She worked in her late teens for the Ladies Cooperative Guild, a Christian socialist organization where she supervised young girls making toys. Through this work she saw the housing conditions in which the young employees lived. She fell under the influence of John Ruskin, an influential art critic and social commentator, who in his writings showed how the impact of industrialism undermined pride in craftsmanship. Hill, like other COS thinkers, believed throughout her life that social work should bring elements of society together, that society is – or should be – a cohesive, organic whole and that the existence of great numbers of urban poor was a mortal threat to this ideal. She wanted to achieve social harmony without upheaval – just as did others such as Ruskin and the young historian Arnold Toynbee.

There are two radically different views of Octavia Hill and her work.

One: That she was a principal instigator of upper middle-class tutelage of the working poor. She insisted that her tenants pay rent regularly, with no excuses admitted. She played down the differences between social classes and called for fellowship and friendship between middle class and working class and preferred to see her tenants as individuals not defined by class. Nor did she advocate change in the social structure. For all her talk of empathy she held the belief very strongly that an individual's character, moral make-up and sense of self-responsibility were the only factors relevant in explaining why some people are poor and some are not. She was oblivious to the effect of the economic downturns, of the labour market in depression and opposed any policies that would appear to encourage work avoidance in the parents and adults – including free school dinners for impoverished children and old age pensions.

Two: That she had a deep faith in the capacity of individuals to change and in particular to acquire different habits and a morality of responsibility. She considered herself a Christian socialist and used words like 'love' and 'compassion' in relation to the poor. 'Our ideal must be to promote the happy natural intercourse of neighbours – mutual knowledge, mutual help' (Hill 2010 [1875]: 15). She had a deep reverence for the unique value and dignity of all individuals and admired those who lived in poverty and struggled to retain their self-respect. In her training of fellow workers she emphasized the importance of empathy and of building relationships. Although she was devoted to the Church of England she did not, as other evangelicals did, provide aid only to those who would read religious tracts of their particular denomination. She also opposed environmental degradation of urban neighbourhoods and later in life helped found the National Trust.

In *Homes of the London Poor* (1875) she wrote that, when visiting families, 'there would be no interference, no entering their rooms uninvited, no offer of money or the necessaries of life'. But she would offer any help that could be given to friends without insult:

> sympathy in their distresses; advice, help and counsel in their difficulties; introductions that might be of use to them; means of education; visits to the country; a loan of books; a bunch of flowers brought on purpose; an invitation to any entertainment, in a room built at the back of my own house...
>
> (Hill 1875: 42)

She also wrote:

> The people's homes are bad, partly because they are badly built and arranged; they are tenfold worse because the tenants' habits and lives are what they are. Transplant them tomorrow to healthy and commodious homes, and they would pollute and destroy them. There needs, and will need for some time, a reformatory work which will demand that living zeal of individuals which cannot be had for money, and cannot be legislated for by Parliament.
>
> (Hill 1875: 10)

Read these excerpts from Hill's *Letters*. Which of the two views of Hill's work do you think is the more accurate? Do you think she would make a good social worker today?

There was more to the COS than the call to reduce drastically outdoor poor relief. The main figures within the Society – Bernard and Helen Bosanquet, Octavia Hill and, early on, Samuel Barnett who later founded Toynbee Hall – had, like a whole generation of Victorian reformers, been inspired by the idealist philosophy of T. H. Green (1836–1882), a lecturer at Oxford University and a central figure in the emerging progressivism of the Liberal Party at that time. Green, in his lectures and writings (most published posthumously), promoted an expanded view of social justice and laid out a range of social and political obligations for individuals that required their involvement in social affairs (Harris 1992).

The leading thinkers and philosophers of the charity organization movement were of the same idealist school as Green. They believed in an inclusive concept of active citizenship and were passionate in their campaign to end human degradation wrought by the market economy. They thought that working people should not be reduced to mere elements of production. In their view the fight for the good society involved a contest within the individual; the poor needed allies for that struggle but not dependence on the state. Yet, unlike Green who outlined a role for the state in social reform, the COS thinkers were firmly of the conviction that, outside the Poor Law, all charity should be administered by voluntary organizations.

T. H. Green and philosophic idealism

Green blended a high-minded devotion to social improvement with a more ag-nostic, questioning relationship to the Christian faith and its institutions. The implications of Darwinism in particular had shaken the standard forms of Chris-tian conviction throughout the 1860s. Lecturing as a political philosopher and preaching sermons at Balliol, Green provided a pathway to undergraduates (and others beyond the university) to realize a higher self: God is within you; act in harmony with your higher self and 'to realise that harmony acts always to pro-mote the common good' (Meacham 1987: 13). Much as communitarians in our own time, Green argued that individuals are inescapably part of society, that they cannot disconnect themselves from that society; they have a duty to serve, and often that service means sacrifice. Citizenship reflects the common interests of the society in which people live – the definition of a communal and higher self. State action is justified when it facilitates individuals in cultivating their higher self. For example, Green supported the 1870 Education Act that gave permissive powers to local authorities to rationalize primary schooling in their areas and to build new schools if necessary; he went beyond it in thinking the Act should have made primary schooling compulsory.

From family visiting to social casework

The COS held the view, widely shared by other voluntary societies and the middle class generally, that poverty was a condition that could be tackled by their direct, personal action. COS family visitors pulled together elements of family visiting that had been part and parcel of practice: casework. The word 'case' was used from the beginning to signal that the work involved a systematic investigation of an individual or family through a set sequence of activities: initial home visit, one or more interviews, investigation of evidence, and decision by the case committee. Increasingly from the 1890s, COS thinkers used the phrase 'social work' to describe the investigation and the help, guid-ance and support that practitioners provided for those deemed deserving of help.

For all that casework was central to its practice, COS founders' writing on casework was not taken to great depth. In essence, it offered a basic story of what had happened to the client – including mishaps, unfolding events for the family and a rudimentary description of character, but without any effort to diagnose a problem. Octavia Hill (1875), C. S. Loch (1910) and Helen Bosanquet (1914) each in turn gave some idea as to how casework should be carried out around the turn of the twentieth century. Nevertheless, several themes that characterized casework until the late 1950s were already evident at this time: (i) the power of a sympathetic relationship to transform the outlook of those needing aid; (ii) the necessity of carrying out a thorough investigation into all aspects of an applicant's life; and (iii) the idea that intervention should aim primarily at attitudinal and behaviour change and give limited, material relief only in very specific instances.

C. S. Loch on casework

Charles Stewart Loch (1849–1923) became the executive head of the COS in 1876 and remained at the top of the organization for nearly forty years. He was chief organizer, administrative secretary and principal mouthpiece all in one. For him, love should be the binding force in relationships and he drew heavily on Christianity when he was discussing the foundations of the COS. But he also outlined the method of the family visitor – and proved a big influence on Mary Richmond, an American who later produced the first major textbook casework (see Chapter 4) when she met him in the mid-1890s.

> The object of inquiry is to ascertain the actual causes of distress or dependence . . . . Two methods may be adopted: to inquire in regard to applications for help with a view to forming some plan of material help or friendly aid, or both which will lead to the ultimate self-support of the family and its members, or to ascertain the facts partly at once, partly by degrees and then to form and carry out some plan of help, or to continue to befriend the family in need of help, in the hope of bringing them to conditions of self-support, leaving the work of relief entirely to other agencies. The [district COS] committee in neither case should be a relief committee – itself a direct source of relief.
>
> In general the inquiry should cover the following points: names and address, the nature and causes of the distress, slight or serious, affecting the family as a whole or any member of the family, the ages of the family, previous address, past employment and wages, present income, rent and liabilities, membership of friendly or other society, and savings, relations, relief (if any) from any sources. These points should be verified, and reference should be made to the clergy, the poor-law authorities and others, to ascertain if they know the applicant. The result should be to show how the applicant has been living, and what are the sources of possible help, and also what is his character.
>
> (Loch 1910)

Discussion point   Mr and Mrs T

The COS is credited with developing the ideas of the 'investigation' in which clients' needs and circumstances are determined and the decision recorded as to the help, if any, it provided. Here is an example of its casework. What would be your decision regarding this couple? Is there a difference in attitude between the COS worker who investigates and the district committee which made the final decision? How would your objectives differ from those of the COS worker?

> Mr. T. Margaret Place, Gascoign Place, Bethnal Green, is a boot maker by trade. Is a good hand, and has earned three shillings and sixpence to four shillings and sixpence a day.*
>
> He was taken ill last Christmas, and went to the London Hospital, was there three months. A week after he had gone Mrs. T. had rheumatic fever, and was takent to Bethnal Green Infirmary, where she remained about three months. Directly after they had been taken ill, their furniture was seized for the three weeks' rent which was owing. Consequently, on becoming convalescent they were homeless.
>
> They came out about the same time. He went out to a lodging-house for a night or two, until she came out. He then had twopence, and she had sixpence, which a nurse had give her. They went to a lodging house together, but the society there was dreadful. Next day he had a day's work, and got two shillings and sixpence, and on the strength of this they took a furnished room at tenpence per day (payable nightly).
>
> His work lasted a few weeks, when he was again taken ill, lost his job and spent all their money. Pawned a shirt and apron for a shilling; spent that too. At last pawned their tools for three shillings, which got them a few days' food and lodging. He is now minus tools and cannot work at his own job, and does anything he can. Spent their last twopence on a pen'orth each of tea and sugar. In two days they had a slice of bread and butter each; that's all. They are both very weak through want of food.

The COS district decision regarding this couple:

> The cause of distress was illness with deterioration of work from three and sixpence to two and sixpence a day, and relapse into illness.
>
> The circumstances are inconceivably ill stated; we are not told the man's age, nor whether his health had always been bad, nor whether he could possibly have recovered and become a good workman again; nor whether he had ever been in a club, nor if not, why not.† In short hardly any of the essential questions which determine how the man could be helped are answered by the statement before us.

But one thing is plain. Had the man belonged to a good club, there would have been no hardship at all, and his health would, so far as we are told, not have permanently suffered.

The sensible thing to do would be to insist on his joining a club as soon as he could pass the doctor. It does not follow that the missing habit cannot be stimulated, and if it can, if in short the man appears curable, then the attempt should be made to cure him.

Now and again a man who does not seem curable, especially after several warnings, will have to be allowed to fall into the workhouse. It would be well to arrange a *very carefully discriminating small* scheme of a farm colony as a more healthy open-air workhouse for these few cases that slip through our fingers, and might, perhaps, be restored to industry.

Source: Extracts taken from the *Charity Organisation Review*, 1876.
*Between 17 pence and 22 pence.
†'Club' refers to a friendly society or provident scheme that would insure workers who contributed to the club against illness and unemployment.

The great majority of decisions on individual cases, at least in the first decade of its existence following investigation, were to recommend that the applicant apply to the Poor Law authorities. This was the intended outcome desired by the Local Government Board, the Poor Law authorities and the COS itself, bringing back deterrence directly into the lives of applicants who, in their view, had grown accustomed to drawing on over-generous charity. In this they were counting on the fact that the poor had been 'schooled for generations into averting the stigmatization of becoming a workhouse inmate and to avoid this ultimate humiliation, virtually regardless of their circumstances, nine out of ten supplicants would decline the "offer of the house"' (Humphreys 1995: 53). In their decision making, unemployment, casualized labour and economic recessions were not considered important factors; drunkenness and immorality were.

On the ground the decision making lay with a 'decision committee' under the direction of a salaried agent who – as in the case of Mr and Mrs T above – would take reports from the family visitors. The latter were virtually all women volunteers, with typically 30 or 40 visitors in number in the provincial societies. Humphreys is clear that there was great divergence in the provincial societies from the best practice models issued by London and that, moreover, the local societies in towns such as Birkenhead or Brighton were small, short on volunteers and had insufficient donations to work with. The national COS conference in 1881 heard that, nationally, casework often fell short of expected standards, with reports 'slovenly and ill drawn' and failing to show the 'real merits or demerits of the case' (quoted in Humphreys 1995: 112).

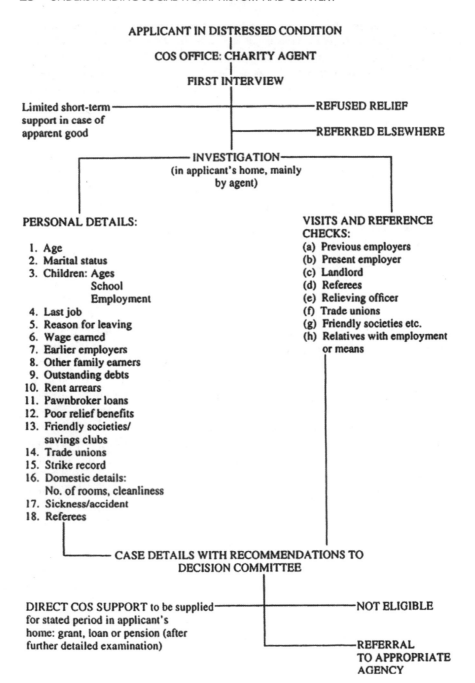

APPLICANT IN DISTRESSED CONDITION

COS OFFICE: CHARITY AGENT

FIRST INTERVIEW

Limited short-term ———————————————————— REFUSED RELIEF
support in case of
apparent good   ———————— REFERRED ELSEWHERE

———— INVESTIGATION ————
(in applicant's home, mainly
by agent)

PERSONAL DETAILS:

1. Age
2. Marital status
3. Children: Ages
        School
        Employment
4. Last job
5. Reason for leaving
6. Wage earned
7. Earlier employers
8. Other family earners
9. Outstanding debts
10. Rent arrears
11. Pawnbroker loans
12. Poor relief benefits
13. Friendly societies/
    savings clubs
14. Trade unions
15. Strike record
16. Domestic details:
    No. of rooms, cleanliness
17. Sickness/accident
18. Referees

VISITS AND REFERENCE
CHECKS:
(a) Previous employers
(b) Present employer
(c) Landlord
(d) Referees
(e) Relieving officer
(f) Trade unions
(g) Friendly societies etc.
(h) Relatives with employment
    or means

———— CASE DETAILS WITH RECOMMENDATIONS TO
DECISION COMMITTEE

DIRECT COS SUPPORT to be supplied ———————————— NOT ELIGIBLE
for stated period in applicant's
home: grant, loan or pension (after
further detailed examination)   ———— REFERRAL
                                                 TO APPROPRIATE
                                                 AGENCY

Flow chart of COS decision making adapted from Humphreys 1995: 113

The provincial societies developed forms of relief that brought stern criticism from London – soup kitchens, provision of railway tickets, providing cast-off clothing and boots, all appeared to the hierarchy in London to blur the line that relief should always be part of a personal plan and be limited to that which was 'individual, personal, temporary and reformatory' (quoted in Humphreys 1995: 116). Cash grants, cash loans and bread were also regularly provided, but the sums were small as were the number of people helped. In Birkenhead, in the twenty years from 1870 the average annual number of applicants receiving outdoor relief through the Poor Law Union was 3,394 and from the COS 444; the monetary value of what was provided was many times more generous from the Poor Law authorities than from the district COS.

The COS and its critics

The COS had its critics from the beginning and criticisms only mounted over the last quarter of the nineteenth century. From local newspaper accounts of its penny-pinching, hard-hearted attitude to specific families in the locality, to more sustained political critiques from the newly born Labour Party (founded in 1906) and Fabian Society (Townshend 1911), the general tone of these critics claimed that the Society was too intrusive into family life, too inquisitorial and too slow and cumbersome in reaching decisions through its district committees. More than that, the COS set itself against the progressive political tide that emerged after 1900. This era of greater state involvement in tackling pressing social problems is often summed up in the phrase 'the new liberalism', denoting the policies that flowed from the Liberal government of 1906 which included the introduction of old age pensions, national insurance and free school meals. The COS found itself opposing each of these measures, returning again and again to its central theme that a person's sense of responsibility must not be undermined. It found state involvement in service provision outside the Poor Law particularly objectionable, such as providing free dinners in schools. The COS, while recognizing the 'fitness of Britain' crisis in the early 1900s (see Chapter 5), would have preferred a children's committee of trained volunteer women to arrange dinners for children in need, preferably from funds raised voluntarily and outside schools.

Bernard Bosanquet on state involvement in poor relief

'[The] commonplace Collectivist treats the community not as a system of institutions linked by ideas and purposes, but as a collection of creatures to be provided for as a crowd, and whose very lives are to be broken up into a series of wants, each to be satisfied as it arises, like the need of a child or a dog. This common tendency is clearly visible in the demands for the endowment of mother hood, universal child maintenance, universal and unconditional right to employment, free medical attendance, universal State maintenance in old age.'

Source: Bosanquet 1907: 14.

The leading COS thinkers constantly wrestled with the implications of their own approach. C. S. Loch himself said in the middle 1880s that he could not encourage people to join the COS, that he had not joined himself merely to cooperate with the Poor Law but for the larger purpose of improving the lot of the poor. Loch also acknowledged the middle-class nature of the organization and he lamented that the aim of following up an investigation of a family by providing 'a friend' was too rarely followed through. He always wanted to rename the organization 'The Society for Friendly and Associated Charity (Lewis 1995b: 61). The COS public intellectuals, particularly the Bosanquets, believed strongly in a cohesive, less class-divided society, one in which the duties and rights of citizenship are conferred on all.

But for all their willingness to look at the Society's shortcomings its leaders and the national organization itself remained adamant in opposition to any state involvement in welfare provision. On this basis it opposed the introduction of free primary school places as well as school-provided meals from the late 1880s onwards, even as campaigns for both gathered pace. They argued that impoverished families unable to feed their children should be relieved by the Poor Law and that where the parents were simply negligent it was better 'in the interests of the community, to allow in such cases the sins of the parents to be visited on their children than to impair the principle of the solidarity of the family' (COS 1893, quoted in Lewis 1995b: 63). On similar grounds the COS opposed the introduction of old age pensions in 1908, as saving enough for old age or joining a friendly society for old age benefits were the exclusive responsibility of the individual and not the state.

Economic circumstances and the unfolding debate about the causes of poverty worked against the COS position. From the mid-1880s onwards, cyclical economic depression, new perceptions of the sources of poverty and the growing willingness within progressive elements of the Liberal Party exposed the rigidities in the original COS model. The sharp economic downturn of 1885 proved to be one such crisis: with tens of thousands out of work the Liberal government of the day urged local authorities to introduce public work schemes to take on the unemployed. Large funds for the unemployed were also raised through the voluntary sector – outside the control of the COS which continued to advocate that only its casework approach was valid in responding to the unemployed. Yet, short of volunteers and with patchy organization on the ground, the COS assisted on average only 800 persons a year in finding work at this time: a miniscule number against the tens of thousands applying for relief.

The COS modernized to an extent: it recognized the necessity of cooperating with other organizations which it had long declared unnecessary since it regarded itself as the coordinating body for charity. It began to convene monthly case conferences to coordinate overlapping work with particular families that it and other organizations were involved with. It gradually admitted representatives from other charity organizations to its district committees, and replaced the categories of 'deserving' and 'undeserving' with 'helpable' and 'unhelpable' and then with the even more indeterminate 'likely or not likely to benefit' to describe those who had been assessed and found either suitable or not suitable for assistance. Significantly, it also tried to overcome a chief criticism – that it was too upper middle class – by recruiting working-class volunteers, a policy that met with little success. It even recognized that in its first decade of existence in the 1870s it had been too draconian in its practices and softened its attitude towards outdoor relief.

Hospital almoners

The introduction of hospital-based social workers in the mid-1890s offers an example of how the COS was capable of adaptation if not fundamental change in philosophy. Virtually from its inception the Society had been concerned that the rise in the number of outpatients attending the clinics of the major hospitals in London was creating a new form of dependency on charity. The hospitals, independent foundations run by boards of governors outside of the poor law, permitted free treatment for those who claimed they could not pay for it. The COS harboured the suspicion that the clinics were being used as a source of free medical care – and regarded the medical charities and outpatients' departments as seedbeds of indiscriminate aid from the beginning.

To save the outpatient clinics their own time-consuming enquiries to see who could pay and who could not, Loch offered to provide an almoner, a COS-trained social worker to enquire into the moral and financial circumstances of the would-be patients.[2] Aware of possible tensions between a social worker and medical staff Loch hoped that the almoner would be treated with courtesy and respect and enjoy the confidence of medical staff. The first appointed almoner, Mary Stewart, was trained by the COS as a social worker and had been employed as secretary to the St Pancras COS committee. She was appointed to the Royal Free Hospital in 1895 with a salary of £125 per year (Cullen 2009).

Mary Stewart (1862–1925)

Mary Stewart's first obligation was to prevent abuse of the outpatient system by those who could in fact afford to pay for treatment. She was to report patients already receiving parish relief, and therefore destitute, to the Poor Law authorities and to refer those who could afford to pay to a provident dispensary which provided health care to those who paid regular contributions. Her duties were chiefly assessment ('enquiry') and referral, which meant interviewing and visiting patients in their home. It was assumed that having concluded her investigation she would refer the person on to other organizations, refusing medical service at the clinic. In essence the role was to scrutinize the boundary between those who could pay or find the means to pay for medical treatment and those who were destitute and were to be compelled to rely on the Poor Law, that is, to attend a workhouse infirmary.

   Stewart had referrals in the first month of her three-month trial appointment, arising largely from the suspicions of individual malingering held by the medical staff. Nevertheless she began to assess and categorize numbers of patients coming to the outpatient ward for treatment. She found that well over twice as many of the outpatients had insufficient income to pay for any kind of medical treatment as those who could. Stewart was only able to interview a small fraction of patients using the clinic in her first year. That proportion grew as with the help of assistants more interviews were undertaken through the 1890s. In essence she discovered that in fact very few people attending the outpatient clinic at the Royal Free were attempting to get a free service they could actually pay for. Only 1 per cent were refused altogether and another 3 per cent told to apply to the Poor Law authorities. Most of the rest she concluded deserved charitable assistance, while some were directed to join a dispensary.

Anne Cummins (1869–1936)

Anne Cummins trained with the COS and then took up a post at St Thomas' Hospital in 1905 is a good example of how hardline commitment to COS principles could mix with forward-looking social work practice. With applicants she stressed the disgrace of accepting Poor Law relief 'unless old age made it absolutely unavoidable' (Bell 1961: 47). She saw herself as patrolling the borderline for the working poor between poverty and health. But for her, the solution was education. The laws of hygiene, the importance of fresh air and nourishing food must be taught – in what today we might call tough love. Cummins, working with both the Lady Margaret Hall Settlement (see next chapter) and the COS, started a centre of social work at St. Thomas'. Windows were opened, wives taught how to procure and cook the most nourishing meals for sick family member; shelters were built for out of door sleeping, and she convinced landlords to upgrade dwellings for tubercular patients. She also arranged mothercraft classes, in which the need for fresh water, proper clothes and rules of infant care were taught (ibid.: 56). Yet on touchstone issues for the COS she remained conservative. For example, on the question of subsidized meals for expectant mothers she said: 'Fortunately this scheme was not adopted. Any movement of this kind would be disastrous to the neighbourhood and would undermine much of the present effort to raise the people from pauperization (ibid.: 59). She believed that every man is responsible for the nurture and sustenance of his own family and that if he was unable to fulfil this obligations he must be helped by others to do so. Those unwilling to make the necessary effort to stand on their own two feet were deemed 'unhelpable'. Subsidizing food for mothers and babies would only undermine the father's sense of responsibility.

Understanding the COS

There is continuing debate on how the COS should be understood within the history of social reform in general and of social work in particular. Two different perspectives, or 'framing narratives', stand out. The first – generally held by historians of the left such as Gareth Stedman Jones (1971) and Leslie Margolin (1997) in his history of social work in the United States – see the main function of the COS as asserting 'labour discipline' by a middle-class organization over the urban working class. This they argue was essentially a coercive and disciplinary agenda that underpinned the exploitation of the urban working class and was designed to ensure that its behaviour and cultural norms conformed to the needs of industrial production of nineteenth-century capitalism. In essence its practice was based around intrusive investigations of individual families in order to assess whether the applicant was fit for work – with the presumption that most applicants were labour market shirkers avoiding their responsibilities. Their argument is powerful and enduring, cropping up regularly in relation not only to the COS but to social work throughout the twentieth century as an instrument of social control and class exploitation (see Chapter 9).

The second perspective locates COS activity, along with moral reform efforts in general, within the growth of civil society as a needed bulwark against a dominant but inefficient state. As such it has greater resonance today than, say, twenty years ago. This perspective takes greater account of the philosophical idealism of the COS, its beliefs in citizenship and the organic nature of society it long held as the ultimate objective of its work with casework as only the means to get there. At the very least, the argument runs, the COS was engaged in stabilizing society, in overcoming class conflict – or at least trying to. Generally this perspective is advanced by historians on the centre-right. They view civil society and voluntary association as immense resources for social support and social concern, particularly when compared with the efforts of a centralized, inefficient public sector. Robert Whelan, for instance, argues persuasively that the COS work was more flexible and inclined to support than we might think. After carefully studying case records he concluded that 'COS workers who...were almost all volunteers, gave a great deal of time to listening and responding to their clients, trying to get to the root of a problem which often lay hidden behind multiple manifesting symptoms, and striving to find the best way forward for those particular people in their particular circumstances' (Whelan 2001: 4).

Summary

- The COS began its work in order to underpin the principles of the New Poor Law and is generally recognized as the first organization to use the phrase 'social work' and to develop the concept of casework.
- Its philosophy underscored the importance of 'character' and that poverty was essentially the result of an individual's failure to accept responsibility and plan providently for the future.
- It also believed that society was an organic whole from which no social class or persons should be left out.
- Its work was carried out mainly by volunteers overseen by paid district secretaries. In the branches outside of London COS practice was more diverse and responsive to local need.

Notes

1. Solly had put forward several other suggestions for responding to the economic recession which sound more progressive to our ears, including job creation schemes for young offenders and the expansion of industrial schools for training urban youth – but it was the concept of more disciplined charity that caught the attention of his listeners.
2. The role of almoner in religious institutions as the person who distributed alms to the poor dated back to the middle ages. The COS thinking was that to use the term for hospital-based social workers would smooth over any difficulties with medical staff. The 'lady almoner' remained the title for medical social workers for some five decades.

Suggested reading

Lewis, J. (1995). *The Voluntary Sector, the State and Social Work in Britain: The Charity Organisation Society/Family Welfare Association since 1869*. Aldershot: Edward Elgar.

Whelan, R. (2001). *Helping the Poor: Friendly Visiting, Dole Charities and Dole Queues*. London: Civitas.

3 The Expanding World of Social Work: Settlements and Guilds of Help

The Charity Organisation Society (COS) had many critics and by the 1890s began to lose its dominance in the world of social work. This chapter examines some of the rival approaches:

- the settlement house movement that developed in part as a reaction to the limitations of the COS;
- the contribution of the settlement movement to early social work training;
- the formation of the Guilds of Help more in line with the 'new liberalism' of the time.

The settlement house movement

Challenges to the COS philosophy arose as further enquiries into the nature and causes of poverty showed that people became poor *not* primarily because of their character but from the environments in which they lived. A range of investigations, some sensationalist, some sober and sociological in nature, revealed that poverty and utter destitution was not always under the control of the individual or the consequence of an individual's poor moral choices. Arthur Mearns, a minister in the East End of London, investigated conditions around his parish and published a blazing account in 1883, *The Bitter Cry of Outcast London*, which sold tens of thousands of copies as a penny pamphlet and inspired a host of similar accounts in other cities. That Mearns communicated his findings in highly vivid language did no harm to his sales; but he also, at least temporarily, lived with the people and within the environment he was investigating, and the element of social exploration of territory that was considered alien and repugnant lent great credibility to his account.

By the 1880s broader questions were also being asked about operation of the Poor Law and of the workhouse system as the principal means through which the absolutely destitute could receive subsistence. Charles Booth, for example, began his epic survey in 1886 of the spatial distribution of wealth and poverty across London. His maps conclusively show the extreme concentration of destitution in neighbourhoods across the East End (Booth 1893). Seebohm Rowntree published his survey of York in 1901 in which he developed the concept of the poverty line. Together they showed that about one-third of the urban population of Britain struggled in poverty. Such evidence undermined the close identification of the COS with the aims of the Poor Law. Questions about the workings of the Poor Law itself became more intense: Should older people have to go into the workhouse to survive in old age just because their working life had come to an end? What about assistance for the sick, the chronically sick and the disabled – were they also only to be given support through workhouse infirmaries? What about children of destitute parents – what kind of education and care would they receive in workhouse?

Partly in response to these various pressures, oversight of relief under the Poor Law was democratized to a limited extent. Local boards of guardians were elected, but up to 1875 all guardians were men. From that date, under pressure from the Workhouse Visiting Society, some women were elected. In 1894 the property qualification for standing as a guardian was removed and in certain areas elected guardians representing the working class who then were able to introduce more progressive policies. (See poster on following page.)

While the COS attempted to move beyond 'the hard and dry years' of the 1870s, a different approach, which would affect social work profoundly, materialized in the 1880s, at first in the East End of London and then elsewhere in major urban areas: the settlement house. If the COS can be said to have been the first organization to work systematically with individuals and their families and to see problems in terms of individual behaviour and moral outlook, the settlement house was the first social work organization to engage in neighbourhood-based work and to attempt to respond to poverty and disadvantage at that level.

Origins of the settlement movement

Edward Denison (1840–1870) an Oxford graduate had 'settled' among the poor of Stepney in the 1860s and argued in his short working life that establishing close personal relationships was the only way to administer assistance and to rebuild community. He too saw 'indiscriminate' charity as a source of poverty, not its cure, and opposed any direct provision of money or meat or bread. But anything other than that could be within the scope of settlers: 'Build schoolhouses, pay teachers, give prises, frame workmen's clubs, help them to help themselves; lend them your brains,' Denison advocated (Leighton 1872).

The first permanent settlement house was established by Samuel and Henrietta Barnett in 1884: Toynbee Hall on Commercial Street in Whitechapel

NO POLITICS.   NO CREEDS.

FAIR PLAY & NO FAVOUR.

MANIFESTO

OF THE

Committee to Promote the Return

OF MESSRS.

J. LOVATT, J.P., H. B. MASSEY, J.P.,

J. BAKER, AND J. BENNETT,

AS

MEMBERS

OF THE

Newcastle Board of Guardians.

DECEMBER, 1894.

Printed and Published by G. Steventon, Penkhull Street, Newcastle.

Election handbill from the 1890s The Local Government Act of 1894 democratised the elections of Boards of Guardians who oversaw the operation of the Poor Law in urban areas. While there had been elections previously – annual in fact – these were often mere formalities with office holders in place for years buttressed by any number of unelected, co-opted appointees. The 1894 Act created three year terms of office, co-option was no longer permitted, the property qualifications previously required for voting were abolished and, significantly, women were allowed to vote and to stand for election themselves. (See for example Emmeline Pankhurst's testimony p. 88).

The handbill here shows four progressive Liberals in Newcastle Under Lyme making a common appeal to the local electorate in 1894. The accompanying manifesto – too long to reproduce here – called for:

- expanding outdoor relief,
- all meetings to be held in the evening so that working men and women if elected could attend,
- the aged poor and children not to have to wear the pauper's uniform if they entered the workhouse.

where it still is.[1] Samuel Barnett had been an enthusiastic member of the COS in the 1870s but became a critic as he recognized the limitations of its approach. Subsequently he engaged in bitter argument with C. S. Loch, head of the COS, who did not forgive Barnett for his apostasy.

The aim of the settlement was to enable university students from Oxford and Cambridge to live among the hard-pressed working class of the East End of London. The Barnetts drew on some of the same philosophical idealism that founders of the COS drew on. Settlers were to be 'as a neighbour to the working poor' and engage in a two-way flow of knowledge: settlement houses were to provide an array of educational and social services while at the same time settlers were there to learn and understand the problems and sources of poverty. It was essentially a form of university outreach into areas of urban disadvantage and a site for what today we would call action learning. The notion of residency was critical to the settlement movement – living side by side with residents in the distressed neighbourhoods of the East End was the only way to get first-hand knowledge of the problems there.

What the Barnetts called 'practical socialism' was not so far from Hill's Christian socialism. It also had its own form of condescension towards the working class: cultured men and women 'who have presumably been nurtured after the best manner in the truths and impulses of the higher human life and the later human civilization' as Robert Woods, an American visitor and later founder of a settlement house in Boston, put it (Woods 1891). Toynbee Hall itself replicated the Oxford collegiate atmosphere: male residents living in male environments in buildings that were built in the image of the Oxford college. In this sense it fitted uncomfortably into the emerging idea of social work as most of the charity workers, family visitors and rent collectors were women.

At Toynbee Hall the social gulf between settlers and the local community was large. The residents, in the early years, were often personally recruited by Samuel Barnett; the overwhelming number were Oxford or Cambridge educated, with many already members of the clergy or civil service. He steered clear of professional charity workers and went for those whom he thought would mix more easily with the people of Whitechapel (Meacham 1987: 45). Although committed to a vision of simpler living the building retained the look and feel of an Oxford college. (Additional residential buildings, added in the late 1880s, were called Balliol House and Wadham House.) The buildings and atmosphere made creating a sense of fellowship difficult. Residents of the East End were of course expected to come into the settlement house and to engage with the settlers. But the pattern of life in the early days of the settlement reflected a cultural hierarchy and local people generally came to Toynbee Hall on its terms and not theirs.

Yet this was only part of the story. Their focus on the condition of the neighbourhood as a whole and as a target for involvement, and their lack of moralizing about character, set settlements apart from the COS. In this context they proved an effective space for innovation and became in effect large social enterprises where adult education classes and boys' and girls' clubs, play groups, infant welfare clinics and mothers' clubs were on offer. Unlike the many faith missions, Barnett, a Church of England vicar, had from the start stressed the ecumenical side of the endeavour: the committee of residents and wardens that set the daily routine included Church of England, Catholics, Nonconformists, Jews, Quakers and agnostics.

Resident settlers were not subject to the kind of strict discipline found in the city missions but were encouraged to do what they were good at in their own way. An 1884 Toynbee Hall brochure outlined the kinds of things that settlers might take up in order to achieve the purpose of the settlement: 'attendance in working men's and boy's clubs; joining in conversation and discussion; helping in entertainments and excursions; teaching on behalf of the University Extension Schemes; conducting men and boys over museums and picture galleries on Saturday afternoons; promoting good music and art' (quoted in Meacham 1987: 53).

From the founding of Toynbee Hall to 1914 some forty-two settlements were established in England and Scotland. At the same time there was rapid diversification within the settlement movement that overcame many of the limitations of Toynbee Hall. Settlements such as the Women's University Settlement in Southwark and later in Bristol and Birmingham were established. They were significant for two reasons: first because women were in the forefront of their foundation providing an avenue for women into the settlement movement; second because they were closely involved in the early development of social work training by offering supervised placements for social work students.

Birmingham Women's Settlement

Birmingham was a city of over half a million residents in 1899. In the 1870s, under the Liberal city administration led by Joseph Chamberlain, it had pioneered municipal reform based on municipal ownership of local utilities – gas, water and electricity – as well as overseeing the paving of roads and the construction of parks.

Civic culture was dominated by Quaker families such as the Barrows, Albrights and Cadburys, and by Unitarians such as the Beales and the Chamberlains. As in Liverpool, this close interlocking of progressive networks provided the seedbed for both the settlement, founded in 1899, and the university, established in 1900. Yet street after street of poorly constructed houses, regular economic downturns and perennial low wages took their relentless toll: rates of infant mortality were high and, in the early 1900s, well above 5 per cent of the population were receiving outdoor relief from the Poor Law authorities (Rimmer 1980: 19).

Birmingham University settlement was founded in 1899 in the St Mary's ward, one of the poorest in the city, by the National Union of Women Workers, which was not a trade union but an organization founded by women working with mothers and children. From the start the settlement focused on the needs of women and their children as they were understood at that time. The founders were well aware of the work that women carried out at home: carding wool, metal polishing, gunstock cleaning, pearl button making. The use of living rooms as dust-filled workshops, the long hours of labour, the participation of children and the absence of any working women's organizations were all factors noted in surveys at the time (Rimmer 1980: 16).

Supported by well known philanthropic families, by mayoral appeals and individual donations, the settlement expanded rapidly in the early 1900s, acquiring buildings and land in St Mary's. The range of activities and services was impressive by any standard:

- A weaving school in partnership with the Crippled Children's Union for Girls who would not be strong enough to engage in the labour market, and a basket-making class with the same aim. By 1904, 168 physically disabled children were enrolled in the settlement. Once a week, residents and students played with the children in what the settlement called 'Happy Afternoons' when the girls would play games, did artwork and heard stories.

- A provident society – a savings scheme through which collectors called once a week, taking two or three pence from each family for banking which would later be spent on extra food at Christmas and purchases of clothes and shoes. By 1900, 130 families were being regularly visited; by 1910 the scheme had been established in fourteen neighbourhoods and five small factories. The collectors – of which there were only nineteen, all unpaid – were to visit at weekends when all family members were in and would often double as good listeners about problems such as unemployment and ill health.

- Worked with the local COS branch to look after widows, older people and anyone in financial need. The settlement was regarded as a source of expertise on unemployment and the causes of poverty and, following the sharp economic recession in 1905, the COS and the Mayor's Relief Fund regularly turned to it for advice and for help in identifying recipients and distributing relief through its numerous voluntary helpers. By the outbreak of the First World War the settlement was used as an advice centre for the locality in distributing financial relief for soldiers' families and for reservists living in the neighbourhood.

- Established a Medical Care Committee whose members visited the parents of children whose illnesses or physical disabilities – poor eyesight, enlarged tonsils, ringworm, poor nutrition – had come to light during school medical inspections. Committee members coordinated hospital appointments, provided loans to buy glasses (and parties to celebrate the repayment of those loans), arranged (and paid for) surgical procedures to remove tonsils or adenoids, and provided convalescent holidays.

- Established Happy Evenings in the local infants' school where, for an hour on Tuesdays at 5 pm one hundred children (boys one week, girls the next) played with helpers who brought games and toys. This was in an era when few households had toys or indoor games. By 1910 seven sessions a week were taking place.
- Ran clubs for girls after collectors visiting families for the provident society reported that girls had nowhere to go after school and no privacy at home. The first club met every evening except Saturday, with singing, writing, cooking and needlework among the regular activities along with visits to swimming pools and an occasional holiday on the North Wales coast. As the girls grew older a senior club was formed; in 1910 a Girl Guide company was formed.
- Working with the People's Free Kindergarten Association the settlement established a kindergarten, with mothers of the children attending invited to classes on child care in the settlement.
- The Poor Man's Lawyer Association was based at the settlement from 1908 onwards providing a lawyer every Tuesday evening for legal advice.[*]

Source: Adapted from Rimmer 1980.

[*]The Poor Man's Lawyer was started by a barrister, Frank Tillyard, at Mansfield House in Canning Town, London, who, although he was a COS hardliner, nevertheless understood that free legal advice for those who could not afford it was essential for justice. When he joined Birmingham University staff in 1908 he brought the idea with him.

By the 1890s, settlements were recognized as centres of action research, a place where social investigations and policy debates went hand in hand. Settlers could learn to gather and analyse social information and feed it into policy discussions. This aspect attracted many reform-minded individuals, particularly civil servants and would-be politicians. William Beveridge, later to author the Beveridge Report of 1942, served as sub-warden at Toynbee Hall in the early 1900s and Clement Atlee, later leader of the Labour Party and prime minister after the Second World War, also spent time within the settlement movement in 1910.

The contribution of settlements to social work

Settlements introduced the neighbourhood as a target of intervention beyond the individual household and family. We look back on the range of work conducted in and through settlements with a degree of amazement that they were able to accomplish so much across so many different fronts. While settlement personnel did not theorize their contribution, wardens did report regularly on the extent of activity: girls' clubs, boys' clubs (forerunners of mixed youth clubs), mothers and toddlers' groups, mothers' education classes, action research about disadvantage in the neighbourhood, lasting initiatives in adult education, advice work, community development work, and family support and home visiting were all part of their ensemble of practice. Rimmer (1980) estimated that the Birmingham University settlement had contact with *almost every woman in its immediate neighbourhood* through one activity or another which even a well funded and dedicated under-fives service such as Sure Start could only aspire to one hundred years later. Nor was the Birmingham settlement alone in focusing on women and on the needs of children and young people. Margaret Sewell led the Women's University Settlement in Southwark from the late 1880s and Helen Cashmore – the first person to obtain a degree in psychology in Britain – established Barton Hall in Bristol in 1911. They continued to be spaces for innovation at least until the First World War and sought collaboration with many organizations. Unlike the COS, which closely guarded its organizational boundaries and only reluctantly engaged in partnerships, settlements were prepared to link with many different kinds of organizations in common enterprise.

Discussion point   Settlement house principles

Unlike other organizations of the time, the settlement house movement thought it was important to live and work in the community itself, alongside local people. Fostering friendships and a sense of equal relationships across class divides and between the powerful and powerless was a major objective.

Drawing on this legacy of settlements, make a list of what you consider to be the advantages and disadvantages in relation to the two points below:

1. To be a good social worker is it necessary to live in the community where you are working? Would your practice be more effective? Is it practical to think that practitioners would live and work in the same neighbourhood?
2. Is it possible to overcome the social class divide between social workers and the people who live in that community? What are the reasons for your position? Would it lead to more effective practice?

Settlements and early social work training

Octavia Hill had long trained her housing managers – and offered that training to others. Young and Ashton are perhaps too generous when they refer to 'the completely new field of social work that she inaugurated', but they do underscore her drive to place the work of her housing managers and COS practitioners on a systematic footing (Young and Ashton 1956: 124). The COS training of its volunteers and full-time staff was regarded as central, and in 1894 the governing council of the COS approved a rationale for training, which included the identification of cases suitable for training purposes, the recruitment of suitable workers and, crucially, acknowledged that training would be useful beyond working for the COS (Kendall 2000: 41). The COS regarded its work as generic and the training which it developed aimed at the breadth of the task as they saw it. At this early point, then, it developed a vision of what social work might accomplish: 'to improve the general condition of the poor in their district and throughout London' (ibid.: 41).

The first significant steps in training were taken through collaboration between Octavia Hill and Margaret Sewell of the Women's University Settlement in Southwark when they proposed a general training course for social workers at the Sociological School, shortly to become the London School of Economics. Sewell had already provided training lectures, practical experience and discussions at her settlement which served as the format for training, and by 1896 a Joint Lectures Committee was formed only to be dissolved the following year when the COS withdrew to form its own training committee. Collaboration continued informally to involve other London settlement houses and COS district committees; the notion of the 'trained social worker', paid or volunteer, was established through an effective network ranging across London settlement houses and the COS (Manthorpe 2002). Nevertheless it was the COS on its own that located its lectures at the London School of Economics in 1903 that provided the first formal university-based training programme.

In Birmingham a full-time course for social workers was established at the university in 1908 with the Birmingham settlement's warden as the lead lecturer – social work training was one of its main objectives when the settlement was established in 1899 (Rimmer 1980). As the University announced at the time, 'Amateurs, untrained and inexperienced, ought not to be turned loose to try their hands at Social Work.... Partly therefore, from motives of philanthropy, partly from the need for real or practical social education, settlements and institutions like them deserve encouragement and need support, and afford scope for the strenuous exertion of good and willing workers' (Lodge quoted in Rimmer 1980: 49).

From the beginning the curriculum was a mixture of academic curriculum and practical learning by attachment to an experienced worker – the staple of all social work training from then on. In particular, training aligned itself with sociology (and 'social science' – the terms were used interchangeably in the 1890s) that introduced two distinctive features: to construct what it regarded as an authentic scientific foundation for the work and to coalesce that work around a set of skills distinctive to social work.

Scottish settlements and social work training

The settlement house movement spread rapidly in Scotland. Toynbee House was established in 1886 followed by a string of settlements over the next decade and a half: the University of Glasgow Settlement, Glasgow Missionary Settlement, New College Settlement in Edinburgh (Church of Scotland), Queen Margaret Settlement (a women's settlement) and Dundee Social Union. As with their English counterparts, Scottish settlements aimed to give settlers the chance to get to know and understand the working class. From the first they also offered training either for missionary work at home or abroad or for social work itself. As the only place where practical experience could be acquired, Scottish settlements provided unstructured, un-credited learning experiences. It was not long before a theoretical component was added to the training. New College Settlement became a centre for learning techniques of social investigation and at the same time acquiring practical experience for which credits were given. At the University of Glasgow Settlement – which both C. S. Loch and Bernard Bosanquet from the COS had visited in prior years – the new rector, Harry Miller, introduced social study and social training (but not until 1920 was a sociology course introduced taught by Miller himself).

For the settlement movement generally north and south of the border it is important not to read back into these first steps in social work training our more defined sense of what a training programme seeks to achieve. Settlements were in fact diverse places providing a range of activities some of which related directly to social work and others only indirectly. Settlement activity became heavily involved in adult education, for example offering classes in citizenship, literacy and history. The settlement contribution to social work training remained almost exclusively practical in nature. Nevertheless this contribution was enormous. They were change agents in training – forming partnerships with universities and offering social science and missionary students access to the world beyond the campus which few of them would have otherwise had access to in the days when undergraduates were drawn from the middle class and largely schooled within segregated social units of their own.

Settlements were (in the main) non-denominational spaces for university men to become leaders; in this, settlements were both gendered and class-based. They were a training ground for those who were headed for the upper professions – clergy, military, medicine, the bar, politics and civil service. In that sense they were a gap filler between university and a settled professional career, providing a means of obtaining a wider understanding of society and rounding out character at the same time.[2]

A plurality of social work perspectives before the First World War

Several profound influences rapidly reshaped social work in the early 1900s and brought it to a point where it could move beyond the contradictions of charity organization ethos and begin to see a wider horizon of activity. These influences opened a more political project for social work by linking an individual's contingent experience to social reform. This coincided with the election of a reform-minded Liberal government in 1906 which for the first time used taxation as an instrument of social reform, introducing in quick succession old age pensions and health and sickness insurance. A new journal, *Progress: Civic, Social and Industrial*, was launched in 1906 by the British Institute of Social Service with a formidable body of Nonconformist liberals such as George Cadbury, Percy Alden, J. A. Hobson and Seebohm Rowntree behind it.[3]

Importance of transatlantic networks

The same books were either published on both sides of the Atlantic or quickly disseminated there or were subject to wide-ranging reviews. Debate, exploring conflicting ideas, imitation, adaptation were all part of the process. The networks were powered by the new liberalism in Britain and progressivism in the United States, both dominant in the years before the First World War. Both movements were broad, political fronts of the middle class that established new ways of understanding poverty and how to counteract it (Stears 2001). The unifying thread that brought them together was the realization that broad elements of social life should not be subject to market forces and that international discussion that pooled different experiences in countering the market was necessary. To this group of thinkers the role of human agency was vital in thwarting the onward march of commodification (Rodgers 1998: 51). This transformation in philosophy and the ethical basis for the good society challenged the epistemological, ontological and ethical foundations of the older nineteenth-century liberalism and 'stripped the market of its trappings as a natural, autonomous and self-regulating realm' (Schafer 2002: 108).

The networks were sustained through pamphlets, conferences, observational visits, exchanges between national organizations, and personal communication. For over forty years charity workers and settlement house organizers were an energetic part of this network. Jane Addams visited Toynbee Hall in London in three successive years from 1887 as she established Hull House in Chicago, like Toynbee Hall a product of progressive Protestantism, though free of its Oxbridge atmosphere (Bissell 2007). In 1890, forty-two American visitors made the journey to Toynbee Hall in London to observe the settlement idea in action. By the mid-1890s American settlement houses had diverged sufficiently from the university settlement concept in Britain to attract English observers who were intrigued by their work with immigrant communities and their links to the women's colleges. The Henry Street Settlement in New York was visited by, among others, Patrick Geddes the doyen of sociology in Britain, Keir Hardie the first leader of the Labour Party, and the youthful Ramsay MacDonald a later leader of the Labour Party and eventually Labour's first prime minister (Rodgers 1998: 64–5). Paul Kellogg, editor of *Survey*, an American social work journal, regularly travelled to England in the years before (and after) the First World War and spent months observing, writing, making contacts within the labour movement and sending regular reports home (Kellogg and Gleason 1919).

Guilds of Help and Councils of Social Service

Although the Poor Law remained on the statute books there was no returning to the principles of 1834 in anything like their pure form. A new spirit superseded the work of the COS, with organizations that, while voluntary, were far more comfortable working with the local government. New civic associations, devoted to social research and the modernization of social service, emerged in Britain, such as the Guilds of Help, Councils of Social Service and other local civic trusts and councils of welfare.

The Guilds of Help brought to casework a broader approach to work with families. They encouraged the development of professional social work, particularly outside London, but at the same time changed its nature by bringing in working-class practitioners to work with impoverished families. Their name was important, using 'help' instead of 'charity' to avoid the association in the public mind with a patronizing and moralistic approach (Finlayson 1994: 170). The Guilds laid a renewed emphasis on friendly visiting but deliberately kept themselves at arm's length from the COS (Moore 1977).

The first Guild was launched in Bradford, a stronghold of the Independent Labour Party, and spread rapidly to other northern and midland cities. Within five years it had outstripped the COS in influence and importance particularly outside London in areas where the COS was weak and often dogmatic in approach. The Guilds practised a form of casework that entered into a casebook full details about an applicant's income, rent, debts and past history together with references from employers. Trained Guild helpers were then expected to visit the family weekly and to keep an accurate record of progress in the casebook. As the basis for that casework, the Guilds stamped on every casebook the ecological chart that Mary Richmond had developed earlier which allowed helpers to map the forces and resources among relatives and neighbourhoods that impact on families (Cahill and Jowitt 1980).

Guild organizers sought to emulate elements of the district visiting systems developed in Elberfeld, Germany, and by the Associated Charities in Boston in the U.S. They aimed to create a powerful constituency for progressive welfare reform by training a large body of voluntary visitors who would raise awareness within public and voluntary agencies for preventive action on poverty. As Moore (1977) notes, the Guilds were among the first agencies to organize community resources effectively; they developed close ties with the Poor Law, and with public health, schools and criminal justice system.

Some critics at the time doubted the significance of the Guilds. In Bradford at least, where the first Guild was launched, although it enrolled prominent Independent Labour Party (ILP) moderates, the local ILP paper, *Forward*, saw it as a little different in impact from the COS (Cahill and Jowitt 1980).

Councils of Social Welfare, formed only a little later than the Guilds, focused on community organizing in a sense that aspired to supplant casework altogether. The Councils were created precisely to coordinate joint working between state-provided welfare through the local Poor Law guardians and charity organizations, and sought to coordinate services in all fields of social welfare by embracing all public and voluntary agencies in a given area, and to promote local programmes to meet local needs. They also campaigned to raise funding, to lobby for legislation and to serve as an information clearing house (Moore 1977; Lewis 1995b). In their most significant departure from COS philosophy, Councils advocated conscious local planning for the needs for all citizens, not just the poor. The first Council, formed by Thomas Hancock Nunn, vice-chair of the Hampstead COS, brought all welfare agencies together under one administrative umbrella in 1902. It met resistance within the COS but by 1914 there was general acceptance that increasingly specialist services needed to be coordinated under a single council (Hancock Nunn 1914).

In 1914, on the eve of the First World War, social work had developed several strands of activities recognizable to us today: casework, neighbourhood-based work, a recognition that families required resources beyond exhortations to acknowledge their responsibilities. The COS was still dominant but had to reconcile itself to the one thing that it had been determined to avoid: entering into partnerships with settlement houses and the Guilds of Help. The Society had long regarded itself as the overarching coordinator of social work (as defined by itself), but by the end of the first decade of the twentieth century found itself with diminished authority and entering into partnerships on an equal basis. It had largely reconciled itself to the settlement movement but had not softened its attitude to the Poor Law, which it wanted to see strengthened, or to any kind of state intervention to counteract poverty. Social work should remain a wholly voluntary effort, in its opinion. Yet with concerns over national fitness (see Chapter 4) and new liberal thinking about the need of the state to provide a national minimum level of social provision, the tide was running against the COS. Other organizations such as the Guilds of Help were more comfortable acting in collaboration with local authorities, and on this major issue – public sector service versus voluntary association – the COS would find itself fighting a lengthy but ultimately losing battle over the next decades.

Summary

- The COS had its critics who asserted that it did not understand the nature of poverty and was too stern in its approach in its collaboration with the Poor Law.
- In contrast, the settlement house movement offered education, cultural events and forms of family support; however, it too was staffed largely by middle-class volunteers, and the social gap between them and those they served was large.
- The settlement movement played a significant role in early social work training, collaborating with the COS.
- The Guilds of Help, based in the north of England, deployed a home visiting system like the COS but saw poverty as a function more of economics than of individual character.

Notes

1. The hall was named after Arnold Toynbee (1852–1883) an Oxford University economist who believed passionately in bringing education to the East End working class.
2. I am indebted to Kate Bradley and her paper presented to a conference at Toynbee Hall in November 2010 for some of the points in this section.
3. Hobson later attacked the COS in *The Crisis of Liberalism* (1909) because it unconsciously deterred its investigators from actually learning from their intended beneficiaries; nor did they understand how an adverse environment hindered the very moral conduct that they sought. Hobson thought classless COS friendships were impossible because its workers could never comprehend the situation of the poor: 'the "case" does not truly reveal itself, because it feels it is regarded as a "case"' (Harrison 1974: 53).

Suggested reading

Briggs, A. and A. Macartney (1984). *Toynbee Hall: The First Hundred Years*. London: Routledge & Kegan Paul.

Gilchrist, R. and T. Jeffs (eds) (2001). *Settlements, Social Change and Community Action: Good Neighbours*, chs 2,5,6 and 7. London: Jessica Kingsley Publishers.

4   Social Work between the Wars

This chapter discusses:

- the political turn to the right following the First World War;
- the work of Mary Richmond, the first to develop a comprehensive system of casework;
- the mental hygiene movement and its impact on casework;
- the importance of gender in social work's effort to become a profession;
- the emergence of the child guidance clinics and the psychiatric social worker;
- the impact of the Great Depression in the 1930s.

War and changing attitudes

The First World War, which broke out in August 1914 and lasted until the end of 1918, brought unparalleled carnage to Europe. Among British casualties some 1.6 million men were wounded, nearly 700,000 killed and another 140,000 declared missing and presumed dead. Following the destruction hopes were high for a fairer postwar world in which the urban working class, having fought for king and country, would find its full and proper reward in the postwar settlement. Public opinion swung against the application of the Poor Law for the dependants of soldiers. A new Ministry of Labour was created to deal with unemployment, while the welfare section of the Munitions Ministry under Seebohm Rowntree was stocked with social progressives (Lowe 1986). In 1918 the new constitution of the still young British Labour Party, *Labour and the New Social Order*, included the celebrated Clause IV committing the party to nationalizing the means of production. There was, however, a definite place for voluntary organizations in the postwar world in Labour's eyes. Sidney Webb, author of Labour's constitution, in speaking to a conference of social workers at the Home Office towards the end of the war described the relation between public and voluntary organizations: 'The Public Authority and the salaried official can only do the work in gross; they are apt to be blunt and obtuse; to have no fingers, but only thumbs.... We need the voluntary worker to be the eyes and fingers of the Public Authority' (quoted in Macadam 1934: 29).

Yet the political landscape soon moved sharply to the right. The new liberalism that prevailed before the war stalled. Long-running labour disputes in the 1920s (with miners' strikes and strikes on the Clyde the most prominent) constituted organized resistance to economic retrenchment and reduced wages, and culminated in the general strike of 1926. Despite Labour forming its first government in 1921 – albeit without a majority in the House of Commons and lasting only a year – the vision for a fairer postwar society ran into stiff headwinds.

From that point on, until the outbreak of the Second World War, Britain was largely governed by Conservative-dominated governments, intent on balancing budgets, cutting public expenditure and in particular unemployment benefits, and supporting employers in their fights with the unions. While the Labour Party again formed a short-lived government in 1929, the onset of the depression quickly restored the Conservatives to power, first in the form of a National Coalition in 1931 and then in a lopsided victory over Labour in the general election of 1935.

Shifting attitudes in the voluntary and public sector

War had accelerated the role of the state, particularly the local authorities, which were enabled by Parliament to provide specific services for learning disability, children's welfare and public health. The Mental Deficiency Act passed in 1913 and the Child and Maternal Welfare Act passed in 1918 were perhaps the most significant milestones in this period of transition that removed large groups of persons from the reach of the Poor Law (see Chapters 5 and 6).

Deeper shifts in public and practitioner attitudes alike were also under way. More and more, the Charity Organisation Society (COS), now fifty years old, was placed on the defensive as it continued to support the idea of an autonomous voluntary sector which, it argued, should not be state-aided in any way. Its willingness to cooperate with public sector services was limited and grudging (Lewis 1995b: 85). But the feeling was mutual, at least among those authorities controlled by the rising Labour Party. A future leader of the Labour Party (and prime minister after the Second World War), Clement Atlee, in his survey of post First World War social work, relegated the COS to an insignificant role because of its reluctance to cooperate with local authorities and for its continued opposition at national level to all social reform measures (Atlee 1920). (It has to be added that he also thought settlement houses past their prime.) Councils of Social Service were formed following the war to coordinate voluntary and statutory authorities in their efforts to relieve distress in ways that explicitly distanced the Councils from the COS. A contemporary review in 1929 by the National Council of Social Service, the umbrella group for the Councils, noted that in those local authorities where the Labour Party was in power, cooperation between the COS and the local authority did not exist (Lewis 1995b: 86).

Other voluntary organizations involved in service delivery, for example in 'mental deficiency' (see Chapter 5), welcomed collaboration with the local authority across a range of services. However this pragmatism, as Lewis notes, left social work in a theoretical vacuum. There was no attempt to develop a theory of charity or social work as a whole, as the COS had done in the last decades of the nineteenth century. Voluntary activity was conceptualized in relation to the state, not on its own account (Lewis 1995b: 87). The immense role that the COS had sketched out for social work – remaking society by improving character and providing moral uplift – was left behind, with nothing to take its place.

Consolidation of casework

While the COS had placed casework on a systematic foundation it had never detached it from its major social objectives – the improvement of character, responsibility for self and strengthening citizenship as the basis for social cohesion. However, thinkers of the next generation of social work increasingly discovered the significance of complexity, causation and accumulated detail that they deemed necessary for good casework and at the same time began to highlight casework as an end in itself. The quantity of descriptive data increased as caseworkers utilized different techniques for ferreting out information that gave their account validity, drawing in the smallest detail as evidence for judgement on family relations or origins of problems. Maintaining privacy was not a concern nor were there inhibitions about asking for information regarding particular individuals from other agencies and organizations – church or chapel, medical clinics, schools.

Mary Richmond (1861–1928), who headed the Baltimore COS in the United States and later in Philadelphia (and later still became director of the Social Work Department at the Russell Sage Foundation in New York), became the first great systematizer of casework with a wide readership on both sides of the Atlantic. Richmond met C. S. Loch in Baltimore when he visited the city in 1895. She later wrote of this meeting:

> One of the cities visited by the London Secretary [C. S. Loch] has been Baltimore, and it was during that visit that I saw for the first time a case record – one brought from England – which marched from definite premises toward a definite conclusion. The conclusion

was one with which I could not now agree, but he made me see, as I had not seen before, that we had been faithfully recording many aimless visits; that the constructive, purposeful mind was not behind our entries.

(Richmond 1917: 5)

In a subsequent visit to England, she was deeply influenced by the idealist philosophy and practice of Bernard and Helen Bosanquet and by the COS ethos of 'love working with discernment' under Loch's leadership (Agnew 2004).

Like the Bosanquets themselves, she opposed government measures for social reform and remained firm in her view that social work should be a sphere of voluntary sector activity separate from government. On the one hand she warned co-workers not to 'permit themselves to be swept away by enthusiastic advocates of social reform from that safe middle ground which recognizes that character is at the very centre [of social problems]' (quoted in Lubove 1969: 11).

On the other hand, she did recognize that family relationships and the environment families lived in heavily impinged on the formation of their character. Early on, in 1901, Richmond elaborated what can now be seen as a rudimentary social systems theory: that the family and individual both constitute and are constituted by various subsystems that link them to wider social groups such as workplace and other neighbourhood organizations. Understanding the person-in-their-situation, which she first attempted to theorize, became the hallmark of casework for the next forty years.

Mary Richmond's *Social Diagnosis*

Richmond's *Social Diagnosis*, published in 1917, provided an advanced handbook read by students for the next two decades. She clearly sought to establish 'social diagnosis' on a par with a medical diagnosis that could only be reached after exhaustive investigation of what she called 'social evidence'. She wrote:

> Social diagnosis is the attempt to arrive at as exact a definition as possible of the social situation and personality of a given client. The gathering of evidence, or investigation, begins the process, the critical examination and comparison of evidence follows, and last comes its interpretation and the definition of the social difficulty. Where one word must describe the whole process, *diagnosis* is a better word than *investigation*, though in strict use the former belongs to the end of the process.

(Richmond 1917: 62)

Social Diagnosis is a compendium of questions for social workers to ask clients. It includes directions on how to conduct the first interview, how to approach the different sources of evidence in relation to client investigation and, in particular, how the casework model should be adapted to particular client groups – what she called the feeble minded, the insane, the immigrant family and unmarried mother.

Richmond urged that written reports on cases contain as much detail as possible concerning a family's background, including finances, child rearing and health, family and relatives, schools, employers, neighbourhood, medical practitioners – with the worker primed for gleaning information from every source. Generations of social work students and practitioners followed her prescription for process recordings (the forms she developed were purchased, copied and otherwise widely adopted), and as a result social workers, in Specht and Courtney's telling phrase, wrote 'endless number of lengthy records, most of them useless, for their supervisors' (Specht and Courtney 1994: 78).

Why was her approach so popular, then? Specht and Courtney argue that the first wave of charity organization social workers were confident that they already *knew* the causes of dependency: a failure of moral character or mental defect, and that therefore the notion that paupers had anything of value to say did not occur to them. For a later generation of caseworkers, however, who did not have these certainties, Richmond advocated a seemingly scientific en-quiry into causes of behaviour for which she provided the pertinent questions and the formats in which the information could be taken down and stored (Specht and Courtney 1994: 79). Somewhere from the mass of information accumulated a proper diagnosis could be made.

The 'psychological turn'

Richmond's articulation of casework was overtaken in the years following the First World War, when social work took a new turn influenced by expanding psychiatric knowledge and the notion of mental hygiene. 'Individualization' became central to social work discourse and, with it, an increasing interest in the inner dynamics of the individual personality. The overarching aim became, not to discern whether a particular individual required particular assistance, but to help the individual to harmonize their personality with the social realities they faced. Those working most directly with these concepts in the field – particularly the new psychiatric social workers in 'mental hygiene' – became the first real elite within social work.

How far the 'psychological turn' actually affected day-to-day casework in the years between the wars has been hotly debated. Woodroofe (1962) described the parallel developments in the United States and Britain as a 'psychiatric deluge', and a positive one at that. 'When it receded,' she wrote in a debatable statement, 'it left rich alluvial soil in which new concepts were to take root and flourish, and older ones were to be vitalized and shaped anew. From these developments, especially from the teaching of Freud and his disciples, there was to emerge not only a new way of thinking about people, but an entirely new way of helping them' (Woodroofe 1962: 119–20). This new orientation would grow in influence, further buttressed by psychoanalytic principles, reaching full flower after the Second World War.

Yelloly (1980) by contrast has argued that, in comparison with the United States, the new orientation in Britain was limited in impact and more pragmatic. In the 1920s the United States entered a conservative phase in politics and culture in which 'success and achievement were highly valued while failure was a mark of person inadequacy. Within this individualist ethos, problems of the social order were given less prominence while psychoanalytic ideas with their reemphasis on the individual easily took root' (Yelloly 1980: 69). By contrast, this individualist ethos was not as strong in Britain while at the same time Britain was well on the road to the public provision of welfare services.

While it is difficult, and probably fruitless, to measure the intensity of this turn across the diverse sectors of social work in the 1920s and 1930s, it is incontestable that by the end of this period sections of British social work had begun to draw on American ideas. In the early days of social work the flow of ideas, methods and institutions, from charity organization to settlements and from youth clubs to casework, moved from Britain to the United States. Now, the flow was the other way, as concepts and practice geared to mental hygiene flooded in. Part of its appeal was that it provided a new language in which to restate the aims of social work as older moral and religious categories were losing their traction. Even the COS found elements in the new psychology to buttress its perspective of self-help and family-based support (Pringle 1928).

Terminology changed. Behaviour that had been ascribed broadly to 'character' before the First World War was recast in terms of 'personality', and judgements on personality now relied on terms such as 'feckless', 'incorrigible', 'deviant'. Those individuals trying to master primitive psychic energies were regarded as reluctant to submit to higher forms of social authority. References to the 'social problem family' became more numerous (Starkey 2000). The new language also introduced concepts such as the client's potential for self-expression and self-actualization, with social workers making judgements on the qualities of the individual personality that either adapts or fails to adapt to the social environment.

In the wake of this new orientation, casework focused more on assessing maladaptive behaviour. A discourse of self-fulfilment and individual attainment detached the individual/client from the notions of active citizenship and the cohesive society that the older generation of idealist thinkers around the COS and Guild of Help workers had long held as the final goal for casework. Two influential textbooks redesigned casework in light of psychological knowledge: *Mental Hygiene and Social Work* by Porter Lee and Marion Kenworthy (1928), and *A Changing Psychology in Social Case Work* by Virginia Robinson (1930). Both were read widely in Britain (Morris 1950). A lecture by Lee, director of the New York School of Social Work at Columbia University, in Birmingham in August 1928 brought out all the COS city directors to hear him emphasize the importance of casework across all forms of social work. In her general account of social casework in Britain at the end of the 1930s, virtually all of Clement Brown's references were to American authors (Clement Brown 1939).

In the early 1920s, technical words from psychoanalytic literature began to displace the earlier vocabulary. In place of the thorough but straightforward elements of sound investigation developed by the COS and systematized by Richmond, newer ideas appeared such as 'transfer', first used by Jessie Taft (Taft 1924), 'rapport', and 'identification', signalling a 'more objective concern with the meaning of relationship to the client and the worker's responsibility in this experience' (Robinson 1930: 129). In comparing social work records from 1924 with those of 1934, Clement Brown noted approvingly the considerable change in language. Whereas the earlier records suggested social work concerns with specific behaviours – 'cleanliness', 'honesty', 'sobriety' – and with material conditions, the later records gave far more detail on aspects of personality, from which she concluded that social problems were more dependent on attitudes and intimate social relationships of the individual than upon 'his superficial habits and physical surroundings' (Clement Brown 1939: 385).

Mental hygiene and the psychiatric social worker

The mental hygiene movement had already seen rapid development before the war in the United States following the publication in 1908 of Clifford Beers' *A Mind that Found Itself*, which is often credited with sparking the mental hygiene movement. Mary C. Jarrett and psychiatrist Elmer Stouthard, working together at the Boston Psychopathic Hospital from 1913 to 1920, were instrumental in the development of psychiatric social work (Lunbeck 1992; Gabriel 2005).[1] While dealing with men with war trauma – then called 'shell shock' but now recognized as post traumatic stress disorder – both had become interested in a wider field: responding to the individual's problems in everyday life that they regarded as indicative of maladjustment (Gabriel 2005). They developed a treatment method based on 'individualization' which aimed to bring the psychologically maladjusted into harmony with the broader social environment in which they lived or worked through the creation of personal relationships that would treat each patient as unique (ibid.: 434). As Jarrett wrote: 'Mental hygiene means individualization above everything; it aims to give free play to the development of the personality' (Jarrett 1921: 364).

In Britain, the psychiatric social worker first emerged in another American import: child guidance clinics.[2] These were funded on both sides of the Atlantic by the American Commonwealth Fund as part of its Mental Hygiene Program. Based on the earlier work of Cyril Burt, the first psychologist appointed to the education department of the London County Council, William Healy (British born but American based) and Adolf Meyer an Austrian psychiatrist based in Boston, the Fund prescribed a model for a preventive, multi-disciplinary team, led by a psychiatrist, that would respond to problems or potential problems of any child. The Commonwealth Fund guided the form that clinics were to take at every step. It funded carefully structured visits to the United States by British magistrates and social workers who, on their return, expressly called for clinics to be set up in Britain on the Commonwealth Fund model. Both the Child Guidance Council and the nation's first child guidance clinic were established soon thereafter, in 1927.

The psychiatric social worker role within child guidance was spelled out in the London County Council's handbook for social workers in 1936: since treatment was seen as dependent on parents' attitudes, social workers were to explain the treatment to parents, convey the psychiatrist's advice and instructions and if needed modify parental attitude. They were also to hold weekly interviews through which parents were gradually to become aware of the role their problems played in shaping their child's behaviour (LCC 1936: 86). The clinics brought a new language to social work – children became 'patients', problems were 'symptoms', causes were 'aetiological factors' requiring 'treatment'. (For contemporary sources on the emergence of child guidance see Lee and Kenworthy 1928; Glueck 1934; and Towle 1941.)

The quest for professional status

Developments in casework were linked to a growing sense within social work of its particular expertise that went hand in hand with claims that social work should be regarded as a profession.

Scope for women's professional aspirations

From the beginning, middle-class women had played a leading role in the formation of social work. Octavia Hill, Helen Bosanquet (née Dendy), Margaret Sewell, Helen Cashmore and others had carved out their own roads to influence, helping to create new institutions as they did so. They are only some of the most prominent. It is estimated that by the late nineteenth century twenty thousand salaried and half a million voluntary women were involved in be-friending and family visiting (Simey 1951). There were many motivations for this involvement – self-discovery, adventure, philanthropic goals, professional development. There was also, as Margaret Simey observed,

> especially amongst women, a doubtless unsuspected dissatisfaction with urban life, an unrecognised need to serve, and so to become part of, an ordered and stable community. Nor can the suspicion be avoided that underneath everything else lay a common compunction at the price exacted from the working classes by the material success of the times. Though the word guilt was seldom used, it was precisely this which was implicit in the relations between the two classes at this juncture.
>
> (Simey 1951: 57)

For women the transition from the benevolent lady visitor to paid social worker offered dramatic possibilities. While it was 'respectable' office-based work, women moving into social work also challenged Victorian notions of respectability, femininity and family not least because they undermined the social status of husbands at a time in middle class families when wives were not expected to work. Yet, while social work offered professional status for women, the bulk of the work was either low paid or remained on a voluntary basis. Moreover, from the 1920s onwards the work brought increasing degrees of supervision and bureaucracy to contend with. Women brought with them the expectations of independence and autonomy from their middle-class backgrounds but had to confront the material realities of subordination in the workplace (Walkowitz 1999). High caseloads and low wages remained common themes throughout much of the twentieth century. These are characteristic of what has been termed a 'semi-profession' (Etzioni 1969), occupations with some attributes of a profession, especially training and an ethic of serving the public good, but whose role is often one of brokering outcomes among more potent participants – courts, medical practices, hospitals, schools and police.

Women social workers in the first half of the twentieth century, whether in the settlement movement or charity organization, had therefore some autonomy and were in a position of power in relation to their clients yet were subordinate both in their own homes and in relation to the wider political and social institutions around them. The large all male bastions of the civil service and government ministries had to be continuously negotiated with tact. While the social work organizations that women pioneers created often attracted members of the aristocracy as patrons, the women themselves were middle class. We rightly consider the powerful advantages that social class bestowed on social workers but it is also important to note that the middle class is exactly that, a class in between powerful and wealthy elites on the one hand and the working class on the other. Its social position is intermediate, and it must constitute itself through material and symbolic struggles, with its own actions and engagements subject to multiple and contested views. Thus there was from the beginning an 'in-betweenness' about social work in terms of its social and occupational standing.

Hospital almoners struggle for recognition

After Mary Stewart's appointment as the first almoner at the Royal Free Hospital in London (see Chapter 2), other hospitals, slowly and one by one, appointed their own almoners although they remained few in number for some years. It was left to each almoner to work out her own system as they faced the basic problem for which they had been hired: too many outpatients were overwhelming the hospitals and those attending must be helped to use a full range of facilities. The task involved home visiting, and to help with this a general agreement had been reached with the COS that any almoner could draw on its workers if needed. Gradually, doctors and nurses came to see that the enquiries that almoners made could deliver information that they themselves found useful. At first this centred around convalescence and relevant equipment, fresh air and proper hygiene for tubercular patients, and working with pregnant women.[*]

Some aspects of the early almoner's role would be familiar to practitioners today, such as liaison with many organizations – nursing homes, convalescent homes, clothing providers, providers of seaside visits, religious welfare societies (particularly those offering accommodation) such as the Church Army and the Jewish Board of Guardians, and alternative infirmaries. The almoner's role was investigative and liaison in nature – she was decidedly not to be viewed as an alternative centre for relief of poverty but would link those with real material need (if so determined) with those agencies whose function it was to meet that need. The almoner, always a woman, often worked alone negotiating new roles and contending with suspicious medical and nursing professions. The need to tread delicately with the doctors was a challenge for these intelligent, ambitious women with wide-ranging intellects and broad knowledge of the social world. Yet year by year, both before and after the First World War, a new social work role was being developed – the medical social worker.

[*]'Lady Harmony', as patients often called Helen Nussey the almoner at Westminster Hospital, wrote about her patients in the *Westminster Hospital Gazette* – about the forgetful, the tubercular, the shabby genteel and the one patient whom she regularly reminded about the importance of hygiene: 'Lor, yes Miss. I never spits without thinking of you' (quoted in Bell 1961: 41).

During the second and third decades of the twentieth century there were regular calls from within social work for it to be regarded as a full-blown profession. Before the First World War, social work had succeeded in shifting representation of the social worker beyond the older image of the 'lady bountiful', and indeed beyond the charity worker as moral enforcer. One of Mary

Richmond's main objectives in writing *Social Diagnosis* was precisely to establish a meticulous, common practice that would be regarded as social work's own sphere of activity with a recognized method parallel to that of the medical profession.

Is social work a profession?

Abraham Flexner, who had already written a major report on professional organization in medicine, disappointed an audience of American social workers in 1915 when he said:

> I have made the point that all the established and recognized professions have definite and specific ends: medicine, law, architecture, engineering – one can draw a clear line of demarcation about their respective fields. This is not true of social work. It appears not so much a definite field as an aspect of work in many fields. An aspect of medicine belongs to social work, as do certain aspects of law, education, architecture, etc.

> (Flexner 1915)

The early social work professional associations in general began on a shoestring with a small number of members and only extended their reach and influence after several decades of existence. The almoners' first steps towards professional association were to be repeated by the different branches of social work in the twentieth century. The first Almoners Committee was set up in 1903 with seven members. In essence it was established to oversee the kind of work that almoners did, the problems associated with it, and conditions of employment. In 1911 it became the Hospital Almoners Committee, in 1920 the Association of Hospital Almoners and in 1927 the Hospital Almoners Association.

The passage of the Mental Deficiency Act 1913 prompted the founding of the Central Association of Mental Welfare (see Chapter 5) and was an exception in terms of membership. It was able to draw in workers from various voluntary organizations already in the field and remained one of the most important early professional social work associations until 1946 when it merged with the National Council for Mental Hygiene (founded 1922) and the Child Guidance Council (founded 1927) to form the National Association of Mental Health (which in turn evolved into the advocacy and community provider of services MIND in 1972).

The new elite: psychiatric social work

Psychiatric social workers, on the back of their psychological expertise, were intent on establishing themselves as an elite. Although subject to the overriding authority of male psychiatrists, their close partnership with what appeared to be a new and exciting medical field provided them with status and some degree of autonomy. Following negotiations with William Beveridge, at that time head of the London School of Economics (LSE), the Commonwealth Fund financed, and dictated, the content of the first training course in psychiatric social work in Britain, the Diploma in Mental Health, at the LSE in 1929. The curriculum, which became the pattern for subsequent training of psychiatric social workers, included the different schools of psychoanalysis, the role of psychiatry in dealing with social and family relations and symptoms of childhood mental disorders such as bed-wetting, tantrums and anti-social behaviour (Stewart 2006). To ensure compliance with its own model for child guidance the Commonwealth Fund continued to send informal inspectors from the United States to monitor the LSE curriculum for some years.

Psychiatric social work established an outsized presence within social work at large – driven both by the development of child guidance clinics and the attachment of social workers to psychiatric hospitals. Yet their numbers, as with hospital almoners, remained small. The Association of Psychiatric Social Workers, established in 1930, had an original membership of seventeen. Its membership was so small in that year that 'it was difficult to differentiate the executive committee from the general meeting'. Its cash balance was 2*s*. 10*d*. (Timms 1964: 161). The quintessential badge of a profession – establishing a register for qualified practitioners from which they could be struck off – would not set up until 1961.

Other professional associations had already been formed and from the beginning, viewed from the vantage point of the twenty-first century, they were caught in a similar contradiction: aspiring to high ideals for their membership and the public they served but without the requisite prestige and numbers to make their rules of conduct stick. The dilemma facing a general professional association of social work is clearly evident in this earlier history: how to embrace a large number of practitioners without at the same time compromising the notion of professional qualification, competence and authorization of expertise by throwing open the gates too widely to include unqualified or partially qualified practitioners. Each of these earlier associations regarded itself as a separate profession with its own self-regulating organization, while wider recognition of professional status continued to elude social work as a whole. Not until 1970, after protracted negotiations, would the different professional associations finally combine into a single entity, the British Association of Social Workers.

Social work and the Depression

The stock market crash of 1929 inaugurated the Great Depression, an economic catastrophe that threw millions out work and seemed to have no end. For the first time, mass unemployment became a semi-permanent, structural feature of the economy with levels never seen before. In the 1920s, unemployment ran at about 10 per cent of the workforce. Between 1931 and 1933 among those who were covered by insurance some 22 per cent of the workforce was unemployed – close to 3 million people. This did not count the three-quarters of a million workers who were uninsured and also out of work. The government's Unemployment Fund from which unemployment benefit was paid, in William Beveridge's phrase 'melted in a moment' (quoted in Finlayson 1994: 211).

Surveys noted the close link between poverty and unemployment: Seebohm Rowntree looked again at York and found that unemployment was responsible for 44 per cent of those in poverty – the comparable figure in his first survey of York in 1899 was 2 per cent. Surveys from the East End of London and Bristol came to similar conclusions. A number of studies from the 1930s, such as that by the Pilgrim Trust, *Men Without Work* (1937), examined in detail the consequences of unemployment, not just on household income but also on diet, health and mental health, in particular noting the link between unemployment and clinical depression. Other studies, such as the Carnegie Trust's *Disinherited Youth* (1943) looked at the impact on young people.

Dismantling the Poor Law

Social work with families of the unemployed and others in poverty was by now a mix of voluntary organization and public sector activity, with the balance tipping towards the latter, if only imperceptibly at first. At long last, when the Local Government Act 1929 came into force the following year, the structure of the Poor Law was dismantled as the old boards of guardians had their functions transferred to public assistance committees of local authorities. At one fell swoop London County Council took over the work of twenty-five boards of guardians, which included running residential establishments providing for 100,000 people (Macadam 1934: 87). Relieving officers in the main became area welfare officers. Given the swiftness of the change, perhaps it is not surprising that the methods for deciding who was to receive poor relief differed little from those of the old guardians, particularly as guardians themselves advised and supported the new committees in their work.

It is important to remember that the Poor Law, however harsh in ethos, was a kind of welfare state – relieving the poverty of older people, widows, children, the sick and disabled, psychiatric patients, the unemployed and the underemployed as additional specific services gradually developed under the broad category of 'poor relief'. Its institutions covered every corner of the United Kingdom. Across England and Wales there were nearly 600 unions, over 80 in Scotland and some 130 unions in Ireland. The scale and significance of Poor Law institutions cannot therefore be overestimated. While the energy and diversity of the voluntary effort in the late nineteenth century and first half of the twentieth century has been rightly noted by many historians, including those who see that tradition as one to return to, it is only part of the story. Substantial involvement by the state – on a scale that no voluntary organisation could ever come close to matching – underpinned that voluntary effort and left a substantial legacy for good and ill, particularly for social work.

The Local Government Act also actively sought to incorporate voluntary expertise in making individual decisions about public assistance by encouraging the co-option of experienced voluntary workers to public assistance committees. It further stipulated that women must be among those co-opted members (Macadam 1934: 91). And with the transfer of responsibility for the means test to the Unemployment Assistance Board, local advisory committees of experienced voluntary workers were established to guide decisions on individual relief. Great hopes were invested in these social service committees as the bridge between voluntary social work societies and public authorities and the catalyst for wider public–voluntary cooperation. One of the objectives – as it turned out only partially attained in certain authorities – was the registration of every family receiving any kind of assistance in a given area – whether meals or loans for higher education supplied by the local education authority, or milk and home nursing from the public health committee of the local authority or services from the Mental Deficiency Committee (see Chapter 5). Another objective was the coordination of family casework to provide specific forms of help to individual families which would discern, as Mary Richmond hoped, the symptoms of the disease of poverty as a clinic identifies physical illness.

By the mid-1930s, thoughtful observers of social work pressed for the formation of local social service organizations that would coordinate public and voluntary efforts to relieve poverty in given urban areas, yet they recognized that the scale of the work that voluntary organizations undertook was small compared to the magnitude of the problem of poverty. The ultimate solution to poverty and immiseration as Elizabeth Macadam, head of the Joint University Council for Social Work Education in the 1920s and 1930s noted, lay outside of social work; it required drastic changes in the economic and industrial structure, and a more equal distribution of wealth including the introduction of family allowance. She would live to see Britain, following another catastrophic world war, attempt exactly this.

Summary

- Following the First World War the largely Conservative governments dominated the political scene with cuts to social programmes and opposition to wage rises. The period of progressive policies of the prewar Liberal governments was over.

- A new emphasis on personality and psychology emerged in social work thinking led by psychiatric social workers in child guidance clinics.
- In the face of economic depression in the 1930s, local authorities became more directly involved in alleviating poverty, often by deploying voluntary workers, particularly in London.

Notes

1. In 1918 Stouthard reanalysed the cases that Richmond discussed in *Social Diagnosis* and found that more than half suffered from 'psychopathic disorders'.
2. The term 'psychiatric social worker' was coined by Mary Jarrett in 1916 to denote the social worker in mental hygiene.

Suggested reading

Woodroofe, K. (1962). *From Charity to Social Work in England and the United States*, chs 5 and 6. London: Routledge & Kegan Paul.
Yelloly, M. (1980). *Social Work Theory and Psychoanalysis*, chs 2 and 3. New York: Van Nostrand Reinhold.
For a visceral understanding of what the First World War was like for soldiers, consult the newsreels of British Pathé News at www.britishpathe.com/record.php?id=73631; for the social impact of the war and the emancipation of women, go to http://www.britishpathe.com/record.php?id=78524; and for scenes of the Great Depression http://www.britishpathe.com/record.php?id=73943.

5 Working with 'Mental Deficiency'

This chapter considers the development of social work services for people with 'mental deficiency', a phrase widely used in the first half of the twentieth century to categorize people with learning disabilities and other forms of what was then regarded as 'mental infirmity' such as epilepsy. It covers:

- the anxiety raised by eugenicists and social Darwinists over learning disability as a threat to national fitness;
- how the Mental Deficiency Act 1913 created the first specialist social work service;
- the first steps towards community care as support for a policy of institutionalization of the mentally deficient.

Note: It is difficult not to be repelled by the crude terminology that was once commonplace throughout much of the first half of the twentieth century. The terms used then drew on and reinforced popular conceptions based on stereotype and ignorance about impairment, disability and intelligence. They were also in their fashion diagnostic categories widely used by those working in medical, psychiatric and social work settings at the time. In confronting the problem of usage Atkinson et al. (2000) balanced the need for historical accuracy against using terminology that today is regarded as oppressive and offensive. In this chapter, when historical meaning would otherwise be compromised I use the term of the period – not to do so would airbrush the ideology of the time. Learning disability, the more balanced term of our own time, is used when it does not change our understanding of the past.

Lunacy and mental deficiency under the Poor Law

Nineteenth-century law regarding mental disorder often blurred the distinction between those with mental health problems ('lunatics') and those with learning disability ('idiots', 'imbeciles' and 'mental defectives'). The Lunacy

Act 1845 defined a lunatic as an 'insane person or any person being idiot or lunatic or of unsound mind'; in the same year the County Asylums Act prompted a vast building programme to provide asylums for those with mental disorders to be regulated by the Lunacy Commission. The Lunacy (Scotland) Act 1857 established parallel institutions leading to a marked growth in the number of asylums in Scotland – including royal asylums and a growing network of district and parochial asylums. Wards within workhouses were also licensed in Scotland. However, up to 25 per cent of paupers and private patients registered as insane (which included not only 'idiots' and 'imbeciles' – both categories of learning disability – but also those with dementia, 'chronic mania' and 'melancholia'[1]) were boarded out in Scotland within the context of a large-scale trend, nationally and internationally, towards institutionalization (Sturdy and Parry-Jones 1999).

Thus, as with the mentally deficient in England (see below), these first steps towards community care were designed to bolster institutionalization, not to offer an alternative; principally the policy aimed to relieve overcrowding by boarding out chronic patients and to keep the rising costs of asylums under some control. In general, patients were placed in private dwellings owned by a suitable guardian in largely rural villages or with relatives – either singly or with others (not exceeding four) (Sturdy and Parry-Jones 1999: 89). Boarding out in Scotland proved consistent – with approximately 20 per cent of those registered insane – until the passage of the Mental Deficiency and Lunacy Act 1913 which clearly distinguished for the first time between 'mental defectives' and those with mental health problems. The former were then cared for under a parallel but different system.

Relieving officers

Relieving officers (RO) had some social work-like responsibilities for 'lunatics' – those with severe mental health problems – in the late nineteenth and early twentieth centuries. They had the power to remove an 'alleged lunatic' if necessary for public safety before any proceedings to commit to an asylum before a magistrate and to place that person under the care and control of the workhouse up to a maximum of three days or 14 days with an order by a magistrate. However detention of lunatics in workhouses was discouraged so it was the RO's responsibility to arrange for transfer to a local asylum. They were also a member of the local 'visiting committee' – visiting patients every six months and receiving full information on their treatment and fitness for discharge. This included arranging trials at home or boarding out. As their handbooks make clear ROs were to act independently of guardians and should they fail to follow procedures scrupulously they were liable to damages personally by the person detained (Dumsday and Moss 1929). By the 1860s, most workhouses, and certainly all the major urban ones, had established separate wards for the pauper insane. While the asylum system continued to expand – huge institutions in Leavesden and Caterham were built in 1867 – it became policy to send only those certified to asylums, that is, those whose behaviour was clearly unpredictable and dangerousness as judged by lay authorities, and, more importantly, by their own relations. Following the Lunacy Act 1890 the role of the duly authorized officer was created to oversee that the judgements of relatives and others were executed according to the law (Berridge 1990).

The Poor Law, then, slowly recognized the 'mentally deficient' as a distinct class of pauper over the course of the second half of the nineteenth century. Those with learning disability often received outdoor relief or formed part of the 'ins and outs' population within workhouses, that is, those who would enter for short stays. Nevertheless, learning disabled people lived in workhouses in some numbers (in part because they provided useful, even profit-making, labour) – up to one-third of the workhouse population in Norfolk, for example – often housed in the sector for older people or, more rarely, in specially built asylums (Digby 1996: 6).

Social Darwinism and national fitness

At the turn of the twentieth century a mood of unease regarding Britain's place in the world emerged as the level of both her industrial and military strength in relation to that of her chief competitors the United States and Germany, was called into question. At the conclusion of the Boer War in South Africa in 1902, fought not by conscripts but by volunteers, attention focused on the fact that the army had had to turn away many would-be recruits as physically unfit – too short, malnourished, under weight – with as many as two out of three volunteers rejected in some urban areas. Among policy makers, politicians and public intellectuals there were related concerns about declining birth rates among the middle class and the unchecked reproduction of 'the unfit' and 'the mentally deficient'.

To get an accurate picture of the extent of unfitness the government set up the Inter-departmental Committee on Physical Deterioration, which reported in 1904, identifying what it called 'acknowledged evils' such as overcrowding in urban working-class districts, 'with its attendant evils of uncleanliness, foul air and bad sanitation' (quoted in Finlayson 1994: 82). It also identified the long hours, dusty atmosphere and high temperatures in workplaces that particularly undermined young people's health. The report also emphasized the bad effects on infants of women working too late into their pregnancies and returning to work too soon, and noted the general lack of milk and nutrition in children's diets.

Anxiety also came from a different quarter: that through hereditary transmission of learning disabilities Britain's national strength was being diluted. It was fuelled by the idea that society itself was only as strong as its strongest members, and that nations, like animal species, were engaged in the struggle for the survival of the fittest. The doctrine was drawn from popularization of Darwin's theory of evolution in *On the Origin of Species*, published some forty years before in 1859. 'Evolution', 'natural selection', 'heredity' were all power-fully invoked by the new social sciences – sociology and psychology – giving them prominent attention and a new formulation: 'social Darwinism'. The introduction of intelligence testing in the early twentieth century was seen in part as a way of determining the extent of mental deficiency among pupils in schools.

The eugenics movement

Running parallel to the Inter-departmental Committee on Physical Deterio-ration, a Royal Commission on the Care and Control of the Feeble-Minded was also set up in 1904 to examine the issue of 'mental deficiency'; its report (1908) strongly endorsed the principle of heredity as the source of declining national strength. The notion that the condition of society could only be im-proved by selective breeding techniques was central to what purported to be a new science: eugenics. The resulting movement attracted a range of notable intellectuals across the political spectrum, such as the Fabians Sydney and Beatrice Webb, author H. G. Wells, as well as academics, politicians and social workers. At its most extreme the movement campaigned for the voluntary sterilization of learning disabled people during the first third of the twentieth century. Some social work organizations allied themselves with this campaign (see below).

Services for those with learning disability

Voluntary organizations took the lead at the end of the nineteenth century in providing services for those with learning disability. The National Associ-ation for the Welfare of the Feeble Minded, set up by Mary Dendy (sister of Helen Bosanquet, née Dendy) and Ellen Pinsent in 1895, and the Central Association for Mental Welfare formed in 1913 in response to the Mental Deficiency Act of that year, applied pressure on government to improve con-ditions through residential units outside the asylum and workhouse and to clarify the law under which those services could be provided. Voluntary orga-nizations were also active in establishing hostels for the 'feeble minded' and after-care services for children leaving special schools (Rooff 1957: 79–122).

There was wide agreement that the mentally deficient should be protected from the rigours of the labour market and from the Poor Law institutions. Mary Dendy wrote: 'We cannot hope to make them good citizens, to make them clever men and women, but we aim at keeping them innocent' (quoted in Thomson 1998: 152). Their care was a necessary and paternal act intended to preserve that 'innocence'. Themes of innocence, helplessness, and need for protection were used regularly in the first half of the twentieth century as arguments against conferring rights and citizenship on learning disabled people. A campaign to restructure services was led by the Eugenics Society and the National Association for the Welfare of the Feeble-Minded and influenced heavily the Royal Commission report of 1908. The campaign's objectives were: (i) to segregate learning disabled people from mainstream society; (ii) where that could not happen, to maintain a system of surveillance of those who remained at home; and (iii) to ensure that they did not reproduce in order 'to stem the advancing tide of degeneracy', as Alfred Tredgold, author of what was regarded as the definitive textbook on mental deficiency, put it (quoted in Atkinson et al. 2000: 184).

The campaign for a Mental Deficiency Act considerably widened the range of impairments deemed mentally deficient. Those with a *less* severe impairment – the 'adult feeble-minded' – were the source of major concern. In Tredgold's thinking, feeble-minded women were considered to be unusually fertile, prone to promiscuity, producing offspring who were below average in physical and mental fitness, with high rates of illegitimacy, while feeble-minded men constituted a large part of the prison population (Tredgold 1908).

Discussion point   Speech by Mr W. Moorehouse, Chairman of the Wakefield Board of Guardians, given to the General Purposes Committee, 1 February 1911

On the General Question of the Care and Control of the Feeble Minded – the most urgent and difficult social problems facing Britain.

On January 1st 1909, there were under care in England and Wales 128,787 Certified Insane, an increase of 2,703 on the previous year, and of these 91.1 per cent were pauper patients. Separate from Certified Insane, the estimated number of Mentally Defectives was 149,628. Of this number it was estimated that 65,509 were in need of proper provision, and of the 65,509 there were 6,990 in Workhouses and 4,700 on Out-Relief.

Those are very sad statistics. We as Guardians know that the imbeciles are not an inviting class. They are often disagreeable in manners or appearance and not too clean in habits. Yet they have strong claims upon us for better care and treatment. They are helpless. Their poverty is not always their own fault. They are prisoners without being offenders, and must stay whether they like it or not. This is the terrible lot we have to deal with.

What are the different attitudes towards those with mental deficiency found in this speech? What kinds of policies would emerge from this kind of thinking?

The Mental Deficiency Act 1913

The Mental Deficiency Act 1913 proved to be the central statute shaping social work services for the learning disabled until the late 1950s. In essence the Act defined mental deficiency in terms of how an individual's intelligence showed itself in the ability to work, to support himself or herself in the community and to conform to social and moral standards of behaviour.

- The Act removed the care and control of 'defectives' from the Poor Law boards of guardians and gave that responsibility to local authorities, which were required to set up mental deficiency committees.
- Local authorities also assumed financial costs for care and supervision but received grants from central government to allow them to do so – a major breach in the power of the Poor Law institutions.
- The Act established new arrangements and separate institutions for those deemed mentally defective who were to be placed in newly established 'colonies' rather than workhouses or prisons.
- It created the central Board of Control to oversee all aspects of care for the mentally deficient and for those with mental health problems, replacing the old Lunacy Commission.
- It allowed parents to apply for the compulsory detention of offspring under 21 years of age; for this, two qualified medical practitioners had to assent, one of whom had to be appointed by the Board of Control or the local authority for that function.

The main thrust of the Act was to codify the process of 'ascertainment' – investigating and assessing those who were deemed mentally deficient. Once a person was 'ascertained' he or she was either institutionalized or subject to supervised home care. The Act permitted a court to appoint a guardian – a suitable person, not the parent, to stand *in loco parentis*, a power little used except in specific areas of the country. Overall the Act had astonishing longevity: it was not repealed until the passing of the Mental Health Act 1959. (And Tredgold's textbook, full of photographs that were not 'positive images' went through numerous editions through the 1950s.)

The Act established a system of control and surveillance in accordance with what campaigners had sought. It allowed local authorities to detain those certified as 'defective' in institutions approved to receive mental defectives. Historians debate whether some of the provisions in the Act allowed for an early form of community care but it is probably too far to argue that this was intended by the campaigners for the Act (Glover-Thomas 2002). The provision for guardianship and boarding out of learning disabled people was only sporadically taken up in the first years of implementation although it was used more fully in the years between the world wars.

Discussion point   The Mental Deficiency Act 1913

The Mental Deficiency Act 1913 defined four 'grades' of mental deficiency:

- *Idiot* – 'so deeply defective in mind as to be unable to guard against common physical dangers'.
- *Imbecile* – 'incapable of managing themselves or their affairs, or in the case of children, being taught to do so'.
- *Feeble-minded* – for adults a condition was 'so pronounced that they require care, supervision, and control for their own protection or the protection of others; Persons who may be capable of earning their own living under favourable conditions, but are incapable of competing with others or managing themselves'. For feeble-minded children, their condition was 'so pronounced that they by reason of such defectiveness appear to be personally incapable of receiving proper benefit from instruction in ordinary schools'.
- *Moral imbeciles* – persons who display some mental defect with vicious or criminal propensities on which punishment is no deterrent.

What terms, if any, would we use instead of the above today? To what extent are social work values realized in our using those different terms?

Mary Dendy (1855–1933)

Mary Dendy, as Secretary of the Lancashire and Cheshire Society for the Permanent Care of the Feeble-Minded, advocated distinguishing between feeble-minded persons and the insane who had separate problems requiring separate treatment. She urged confinement of the feeble-minded in separate colonies and established the Sandlebridge Colony in Cheshire in 1902. Sandlebridge was the first institution of importance to be certified under the Elementary Education (Defective and Epileptic Children) Act 1899. (Taken over by Cheshire County Council in 1941 as a 'subnormality hospital', it continued in existence until 1989.) She also advocated that the feeble minded should be prevented from having children for the good of the race. She thought the more 'nearly normal' a person was, the more important it was to prevent them having children to forestall society reaching a tipping point of degeneracy.

The Mental Deficiency Act required at least one woman to be appointed commissioner on the Board of Control. Dendy was appointed as the result of her work at the Sandlebridge Colony. She was committed to the policy of segregation and regarded continued residence in the community of those ascertained as 'defective' as undesirable. But she disliked the bureaucracy and the steady round of visiting she had to undertake as a member of the Board of Control. She also faced prejudice as a woman within the male-dominated civil service that regarded her gender as a reason not to take the Board of Control seriously, suspecting that women appointees would maintain their connection with the voluntary activity in which they were engaged.

Dendy provides a good example of the mix of attitudes and perspectives that to our mind are contradictory. She was well aware that 'feeble-minded' women were often victims of male sexual predators but argued that this undermined the race and urged compulsory detention of such women. When she was on the Manchester Board of Education, before being appointed to the Board of Control, she lobbied hard for the creation of special schools for learning disabled children. Yet she described the removal of the feeble-minded children into 'permanent care' as a form of 'scientific morality' that would benefit both society and the individual by decreasing the suffering of the children themselves and preventing future deterioration of the race.

Source: Jackson 2004.

Both the campaign for the Act and the Act itself were based on the assumption that government, local authority and voluntary service provision would work closely together – a very different ethos from the one that had governed poor relief. The Board of Control had a degree of independence from civil service and government oversight that was new in welfare provision in Britain. It was a new type of government agency formed around a specific group of clients and based on specialist expertise, and it proved a model for specialization within government. Services were the product of an alliance between state and the voluntary organizations in the field led by an interlocking network of personnel and financial assistance (Thomson 1998). Government needed the voluntary organizations to help shape public opinion, a task for which civil servants had little taste. An annual grant from government to the Central Association for Mental Welfare throughout the 1920s allowed it to establish local groups.

Segregation: the growth of colonies

The broad consensus reflected in the Royal Commission report (known sometimes as the Radnor Report) and in those campaigning for the Mental Deficiency Act was that learning disabled people needed to be kept separate from mainstream society. This would be in the best interest of those 'defectives', who needed assistance and discipline, and at the same time protect society. The preferred means for this was the colony, regarded then as more humane and more efficient than the asylum, workhouse or hospital. The argument for colonies was thus cast in medical and therapeutic terms: a tool of re-education and discipline rather than punishment. In particular, British observers who visited model colonies in the United States and Belgium based on cottages and creation of a 'village' atmosphere were persuasive in the argument that this was a new form of care institution.

There were, however, other models of care, and as the cost of running asylums rose, and as the numbers of 'feeble-minded' people was rapidly revised upwards, this prompted a search for alternatives. Small voluntary hostels, refuges for 'feeble-minded girls', and small specialized institutions based on 'grade' of deficiency in London were all available options in Britain. There was also the option of boarding out people. This had been regular practice in Scotland with farmers who drew a small stipend to supplement their income. Whole villages became in effect informal colonies – but lack of medical oversight meant that opposition from the medical profession in England to adopting this model was assured.

Despite the pressure for segregation, the colony model was not widely adopted in England and Wales. By definition, mental defectives were 'incurable' and this was central to diagnosis, but psychiatrists involved themselves only with those regarded as potentially curable. Most colonies, then, remained under non-medical authority, and without the medical profession the system remained largely a custodial one. In that sense colonies were little different in essence from the asylums and workhouses they replaced. However, they did alter the scale of accommodation and made the segregation of those with learning disability more acceptable to the political authorities and to the public at large.

Social workers and mental deficiency

Social workers were first employed in the field to carry out the duties laid on the local authorities by the 1913 Act. While the duty to 'ascertain' lay with the local authority the Act prominently encouraged involvement from voluntary organizations, and it was as employees of these organizations that these social workers emerged. The Central Association for the Care of Mental Defectives (soon to change its name to Central Association of Mental Welfare, CAMW) was asked by the Board of Control to execute its policy. Unlike the Charity Organisation Society, CAMW, coaxed into being by government, was already primed to engage with local authorities. Indeed, about half of its executive committee was made up of representatives from central and local government, with local district committees also drawing on local government officials.

Evelyn Fox (1874–1955)

Evelyn Fox established the CAMW in 1913 on a shoestring – a typewriter and £10. Her experience was not extensive either in voluntary organizations or in work with the learning disabled. She had become interested in social work and trained at the Women's University Settlement in Southwark only five years before, and then, seeing the possibilities in the Royal Commission's report on the feeble-minded, kept her eye on developments. She had no great allegiance to the older ethos of the voluntary sector that viewed state intervention with suspicion and had no difficulty in working closely with government. Equally, because of her limited training she distanced herself from those who were seeking to secure professional status through psychiatric social work (see Chapter 4). She led the organization she established for some thirty years and dominated social work in this field.

Fox thought that work with learning disabled people rested not primarily on psychiatric expertise but on experience, local knowledge and sympathy. She wrote:

> The social adaptation of a defective, the study of his own limitations, the correlation of that study with his environment, his home conditions, the further consideration of his employability, the finding of a suitable environment for him if he can remain in the community . . . this is not work that can be carried on in a few moments or by one or two casual visits. It requires the most careful investigation and study, and it requires also that fundamental, real knowledge of the social conditions of the area in which the defective is living.
>
> (Fox 1929: 72)

Fox lobbied for a eugenics policy in relation to mental deficiency over many years, calling in particular for a statute permitting voluntary sterilization. She only reluctantly abandoned the campaign with the onset of the Second World War as popular enthusiasm for eugenicist policies rapidly diminished at the end of the 1930s.

The social work tasks in relation to work under the 1913 Act were fragmented and dispersed over a range of paid and unpaid staff. Referral came from any one of several sources: parents, voluntary organizations, magistrates courts, hospitals and schools (which were the most numerous). The decision then was to 'ascertain' whether that person fell within the terms of the Act. The individual was given a medical examination (in London this was carried out at County Hall) to establish whether they were 'defective'. The Act required that mental deficiency be established before age 18.

A social worker then enquired into family circumstances. In regulations published in 1935 by the London County Council, the social worker, in carrying out an inspection of family circumstances, was to have regard to:

- the nature and degree of his mental defect;
- the mode of living and domestic circumstances, particularly the care and control, of the person;
- the circumstances of his parents.

The social worker was then to compile a social history which included observations on prenatal history, school history and educational attainment, any employment, whether the person is able to look after themselves, whether they were in moral danger, the status and character of the family, and the person or family's financial circumstances.

Supervision

If the social worker ascertained the person as defective, the individual was placed in an institution or under some form of supervision in which they were visited by social workers or approved visitors – once a month at a minimum, more often if the situation warranted it. If the person was removed to an institution, home visits by the social worker still continued, to assess if standards had improved sufficiently to allow the person's return, and to collect a financial contribution for the institutional care being provided. If the ascertained person remained at home under supervision, social workers or the visitors evaluated the standard of home care, financial circumstances, physical and moral environment of the home, the hereditary history of the family and the behaviour of the person concerned. The central question they had to answer was whether the care and control at home were sufficient.

There were contradictions in this role. On the one hand, the Board of Control asked that the social worker as supervisor become a 'trusted friend', but on the other hand the role required the worker to carry out inspectorial tasks in which any measures of support were clearly subordinate. There was also an evident difference in social class between worker and family. In the files of cases left from the London County Council there is no record of material assistance ever provided.

It is important to remember that the providers of the social work service with learning disabled people came from several bodies: the Mental After Care Association (surviving to this day as Together), the Central Association of Mental Welfare already mentioned, the COS, National Association of the Feeble-Minded and the London Association for the Care of the Mentally Defective were all active in the field. None, of course, were employed by the Board of Control but all worked in collaboration with local authorities to carry out the Board's objectives.

In addition to the social workers from the voluntary organizations, trained magistrates, the clerk to these justices (who received all the official communications regarding individuals), enquiry officers from the local authority, trained lay visitors (usually men, and some women from the ranks of the upper professions who did the great bulk of home visiting), Medical Officers of Health, superintendents of the institutions to which people were sent, and of course the Board of Control itself, all were involved in the decision to ascertain a person and in the monitoring of what was happening to the patient. From the client's point of view this ecology of the powerful must have seemed completely bewildering. No wonder with this fragmentation of decision making that people were lost in the system, with tragic consequences (see box on Herbert Connor below).

Social work practice in London was in advance of that of the rest of the country, particularly after the London County Council (LCC) brought these disparate activities inside the local authority in 1930. The LCC handbook for its social workers in the field suggested that essential characteristics for the work were tact, sympathy, patience and ability to see the problem from parents' point of view (LCC 1936). Winning the confidence of parents was essential, as was frankness, in order to allay the anxiety of parents who feared removal of their offspring if ascertained as mentally deficient. If institutional care was likely to be required, that fact had to be faced and its implications explained.

The LCC appointed women inspectors to carry out the ascertainment of individuals under medical supervision, and to decide which persons should be cared for in institutions or to be looked after at home. The voluntary London Association of Mental Welfare provided supervision at home. After 1930 the work of that association was brought into the LCC's public health department but remained divided: the inspectors engaged in statutory work, that is, assessing people's capacities, while psychiatric social workers supervised those persons who remained at home after being ascertained.

Ellen Pinsent (1866–1949)

Ellen Pinsent replaced Mary Dendy on the Board of Control in 1914 and proved more at home within the bureaucracy and administrative tasks. She was the first woman councillor in Birmingham and understood how local government worked. Like Dendy she brought connections to voluntary organizations and publicists for the cause. A lecture in Cambridge during the campaign for the 1913 Act led to the founding of an association for mental welfare in the city for which her daughter, Hester, became one of the first secretaries.* Pinsent established strong lobbying networks with eugenicists, including with leading members of the Darwin family in particular and close ties with the CAMW.

*Today, under her married name, Hester Adrian is more widely recognized than her mother. Hester's own work with learning disabled people through the middle decades of the twentieth century repudiated the eugenicist views of her mother and focused on developing progressive forms of care.

Herbert Connor

The following case study of supervision of a learning disabled person is taken verbatim from the case history in the Greater London Record Office.

Herbert C. – imbecile but admitted under Albert O'Connor (known as Bertie Antinelli) with foster parents – Mr. Antinelli had died, foster mother blind.

[The London Association for the Care of the Mentally Defective social worker reported on Herbert as of 4 July 1919]:

As a child he suffered from frequent fits but seems to have outgrown them, and now has had none for about 3 years. He attended Middlesex hospital as a child of 2 years for about 4 years for fits. The foster mother says he has no immoral tendencies, but is too innocent and has not much idea of modesty at home. She does not let him out in the street alone and he is evidently afraid of other boys.

He is said to be intensely musical, can play anything he hears, and on several instruments and composes a little. He is very useful to his foster father in his trade and he said he would be worth 22/- to 25/- to a shop of the same kind. . . .

The boy appears simple, harmless and has certain aptitudes, but having regard to his immature character and nervous tendencies he will never fend for himself, and is likely to be an easy prey to unscrupulous persons. He is not with his own parents, and there seems no doubt that if his present protected condition were to alter he would at once be an urgent case for Institutional care.

[In March of 1934 the record says]:

Herbert was found to be neglected and conveyed to Caterham hospital as a place of safety.

[As of 11 April 1934]:

His mentality is that of an eight year old boy. He was unable to repeat 5 numbers, nor could he form a simple sentence bringing in three simple words. His reasoning powers are completely absent and he was unable to appreciate the question if set in the form of a simple problem. He was unable to do correctly little money sums. He is obviously in need of care and protection in his own interest.

He is simple-minded and garrulous and his conversation is inclined to be irrelevant. His weakness in verbal association is shown by his inability to give rhymes. He can tell the time but fails with fast clock. His reasoning is childish. He is quite unable to compete on equal terms with his fellows and is of the type that needs care and control.

There are then no further records except one brief entry in 1936 indicating he remained in institutional care. Twenty-two years later, on 23 December 1958, Herbert was 'discharged – but retained informally' at the hospital.

Source: Case notes from GLRO MXS/B/19/04/001.

Herbert's story underscores some of the important aspects of the operation of the Mental Deficiency Act 1913. The reports were written by voluntary visitors who had little training. We can pick up the kind of basic tests that were used to determine the degree of deficiency; we also note the concern for possible immoral behaviour. His abilities – that he was musical and was able to assist his foster father, who was an instrument maker, in his workshop – are noted but make no impact on the overall assessment. This declares that Herbert lacks the capacity to reason and will need protection for the rest of his life. At no point is there any plan or indication of how long he should remain in his institution. In fact the visitors' reports stop and he remains within the institution for the rest of his life.

Discussion point   Working with the 'mentally defective'

Note the terminology and the frequency and type of contact that Herbert Connor's family had. How would services for the learning disabled today contrast with the services that this family received?

Mental deficiency and women

Mental deficiency in women was often associated with sexual conduct. This apparent lack of control over sexualized behaviour regularly led to ascertainment by the authorities – and to long-term institutionalization. The consequence, Thomson (1998) observed, was that 'feeble-minded' women – those with mild learning disability – who had originally been seen as needing protection were now thought of as a source of danger. Cyril Burt, an influential child psychologist of the time, claimed a high proportion of prostitutes (over 12 per cent) were 'dull and backward', which he linked to the broader problem of lack of control over sexual instincts among the working class generally. In particular, there was thought to be a strong association between mental deficiency and prostitution, and local authorities were encouraged to pay special attention to any defective who associated with, or was, a prostitute.

This was not simply a fear of illegitimacy but a heightened anxiety about women's sexuality. A discourse in which unmarried women had to be protected against moral vice was overtaken, at least in relation to women with learning disability, by the notion that individual females were a threat to the community through sexual misconduct and degeneration (Atkinson et al. 1997).

Expansion of services in the community: supervision and guardianship

The colony system proved expensive, and enthusiasm for it waned in the inter-war years adding persuasive argument for more supervision in the community. The Board of Control first used the term 'community care' in 1930. The different ways that learning disabled people could be supervised in the community included licence from a colony, or under statutory or voluntary supervision. In 1939 some 40,000 persons were on statutory supervision, while some 26,000 were on voluntary supervision – in total more than were living in institutions (Thomson 1998: 154–5). At this point, institutions and 'community care' were not viewed in opposition to each other but as linked strategically and ideologically in the sense that surveillance was a prime objective and the welfare of the person secondary (Atkinson et al. 1997).

There was also provision under which legal responsibility for ascertained defectives was given to a named guardian who was paid a fee and, in return, provided a suitable home. The number of learning disabled people with a guardian remained small by comparison with those on supervision – some five thousand by the end of the 1930s. Disputes emerged around notions of best practice. For example, the Guardianship Society in Brighton in the 1920s systematically pursued guardianships for learning disabled people so that they could remain with their families. The Society's commitment to non-institutional care offered a different philosophy and was opposed by the Board of Control although it did not oppose guardianships per se. Despite this, many of the leading voluntary organizations involved in the field drew on the Society's services as the limitations of the colony system – both its institutional ethos and high costs – became clearer (Westwood 2007). Other features of what we would associate with community care emerged in the 1930s. The Mental Deficiency (Amendment) Act 1927 required local authorities to provide occupation and training for those who fell within the terms of the Act. This provision stimulated the growth of specialized workshops and occupation centres and some voluntary efforts to create sheltered employment beyond.

Historians debate how far the practices of the 1930s foreshadowed later community care policies. The Mental Deficiency Act 1913 aimed to protect the learning disabled person from the community – and vice versa. On the one hand, the Act acknowledged the threats to learning disabled people arising from bad environments, poor home conditions, and unresponsive, ignorant, uncaring parents. On the other hand, supervision was essentially a task of surveillance, to monitor the behaviour of the mentally deficient and to protect the moral and physical health of the community rather than to provide any material aid to counteract environmental pressures or to forestall admission into an institution.

The question of citizenship

In the professional culture that developed in the wake of the Mental Deficiency Act 1913 the notion of citizenship was used to define what was *not* obtainable by learning disabled people. They were deemed incapable of engaging in the reciprocal contract expected of full citizens – enjoying the rights of citizens in return for fulfilling the responsibilities of citizens. And because parents were themselves regarded in an ill-defined way as genetically linked, they were not given the chance to take on meaningful partnership with service providers. This was a powerful legacy that endured for decades. It would require an enormous joint effort from disability lobby groups, academic researchers and committed professionals to change both public opinion and policy and practice – an effort that only gained critical mass in the 1970s.

First steps towards a more progressive ethos

One of the themes of this book is that a change of direction overtakes social work (as with other professional fields) suddenly and in unexpected ways. Even before the Second World War Britain was moving away from the voluntary organizational basis for service provision, and services for learning disability were part of that move. Local authorities took over mental welfare work in the 1930s, epitomized by what was regarded at the time as the best practice standard set by the London County Council's work. Within CAMW a more professional young guard emerged which challenged the old voluntary ethos and the cosy relationship that existed between CAMW and the Board of Control. CAMW did evolve; it developed specialized services to sell to local authorities – to provide guardians, occupation centres, national training courses, holiday camp schemes. Not only did it push for greater professionalism of practice but it also vigorously opposed its own organization's advocacy of voluntary sterilization. By the end of the 1930s the majority of its staff became paid professionals themselves, with the organization's main income drawn from local and central government and the campaign for sterilization quietly laid to rest.

Thomson observes that as progressive forms of mental welfare, such as child guidance and psychotherapy, were adopted, working to a partnership model in dealing with clients became the preferred way to regulate the boundaries of normality. This, he suggests, removed much of the anxiety that had previously fuelled the mental deficiency movement as its eugenicist and disciplinary enthusiasms faded away (Thomson 1998: 172). But while the worst excesses faded, the Mental Deficiency Acts of 1913 and 1927 remained on the statute books; learning disabled people were still referred to as mental defectives and Alfred Tredgold's textbook on mental deficiency continued through innumerable editions right through the 1950s. The Board of Control itself was not disbanded until passage of the Mental Health Act 1959.

*   *   *   *

From the vantage point of the twenty-first century we can see that by the end of the 1930s social work beginning to understand that in relation to learning disabled people there were issues of inclusion (rather than segregation) and of citizenship to address. While the 'psychiatric turn' discussed in Chapter 4 undoubtedly channelled social work practice more deeply into matters of personality, family relationships and individual behaviours, it also enabled practitioners to see the moral content and inherent branding and stigmatization that went hand in hand with the terminology associated with mental deficiency. The terminology that came to replace it in the 1960s – 'mental handicap', 'normality' and 'subnormality', 'high-grade' and 'low grade' – would itself in time appear to be degrading.[2] But in its own way it was attempting to remove moral judgement implicit in the old terminology associated with the Mental Deficiency Act 1913. At the very least it marked a small step towards a clearer understanding of what full citizenship means – even if in our view today it was a small step with a long way still to travel.

By 1939 social work with adults was spread across a range of paid and unpaid volunteer staff and across the public and voluntary sectors (see Figure 5.1). The year 1930 proved a key point of transition when substantial numbers of Poor Law personnel, previously employed by boards of guardians, were transferred to local authorities who then became responsible for their employment. Although this was a transfer within the state sector it marked the beginning of the association of social work with local authorities.

	PUBLIC SECTOR	VOLUNTARY SECTOR
PAID	Relieving officers (from 1930 Area Welfare Officers)	Central Association for Mental Welfare staff
	Duly authorised officers (overseeing admission to psychiatric hospitals)	Psychiatric social workers in voluntary hospitals
	Psychiatric social workers (in London after 1930) engaged in psychiatric units and family visiting after patient discharge	Charity Organisation Society officers
		Almoners in voluntary hospitals
		Organisers of Councils of Social Welfare
	Investigators of old age pension claims	Settlement workers
	Probation Officers	Moral welfare workers with unmarried mothers
UNPAID	Tuberculosis Care Committees	Charity Organisation Society volunteers visiting older people, unemployed
	Advisory Committee voluntary workers (with Employment exchanges helping people into work)	Settlement volunteers
	Local War Pensions committees (up to 1918) helping to find work and organise war pensions	Moral welfare volunteers

Figure 5.1 Social work services for adults on eve of the Second World War

Summary

- Services, largely provided by voluntary organizations for those 'ascertained' as mentally deficient, were among the first to separate from the Poor Law.
- Following the Mental Deficiency Act 1913 a comprehensive system for identifying and supervising those considered mentally deficient relied on a combination of institutionalization and surveillance in the community.
- Learning disabled women were often institutionalized as they were thought to be prone to promiscuity.
- Eugenicist thinking, which fed anxieties about national fitness, was dominant until the late 1930s when a new sense of professionalism based on emerging local authority practice challenged the old eugenicist ideas.

Notes

1. We would recognize those last two as bipolar disorder and depression.
2. The author remembers very clearly these words in common usage by social workers and educational psychologists when he began as a social worker in Cheshire in the late 1970s.

Suggested reading

Scull, T. (1982). *Museums of Madness: The Social Organization of Insanity in the 19th Century*. Harmondsworth: Penguin.

Thompson, M. (1998). *The Problem of Mental Deficiency: Eugenics, Democracy, and Social Policy in Britain c.1870–1959*. Oxford: Clarendon Press.

Welshman, J. and J. Walmsley (eds) (2006). *Community Care in Perspective: Care, Control and Citizenship*. Basingstoke: Palgrave Macmillan.

6 The Welfare of Children

This chapter discusses how social work services for children and families gradually escaped the Poor Law system. It examines:

- how resistant to outside intervention the nineteenth-century family was;
- Poor Law services for impoverished children;
- the role of voluntary organizations in responding to child abuse and child malnourishment;
- the significance of the Children Act 1908;
- the beginnings of state intervention in family life, in particular around boarding out and adoption;
- work with young delinquents.

The nineteenth-century family

The legal context of the nineteenth-century family is critical to understanding why the welfare of children only slowly became a concern for Victorian moral reformers compared with, for example, the response to animal cruelty. (The Royal Society for the Prevention of Cruelty to Animals was founded in 1824 but another sixty years would pass by before a similar organization was created to prevent cruelty to children.) Child welfare was entangled with how far the state should intrude into family life, by what means children should be protected from their parents by an outside authority and the extent of responsibility that mothers alone should bear.

The family was considered a sphere of inviolate privacy; one, moreover, in which the rights of fathers were not just dominant but total. In the early nineteenth century across the nations of the British Isles, women as mothers had no legal rights to their children. Both were considered the legal property of the husband. Divorce was rare, difficult and expensive to obtain, available only through inaccessible ecclesiastical courts or private Acts of Parliament. The

Matrimonial Causes Act 1857 permitted divorce proceedings to be adjudicated in court (rather than through Act of Parliament), but still heavily favoured fathers in setting a double standard in law: men could seek divorce on proof of the wife's adultery whereas women had to prove both an act of adultery *and* an act of cruelty on part of the husband.

Children and the Poor Law

The Poor Law system did not pay specific attention to the way children should be treated or accommodated in workhouses, yet children made up half the workhouse population. (In 1839, out of a total workhouse population of 97,000 nearly 43,000 were children.) Under the original classification, females under 16 were categorized as 'girls' and males under 13 as 'boys'. Children under 7 formed a separate class who could, if deemed 'expedient', accompany their mothers in the female quarters of the workhouse; otherwise children were accommodated in the general wards according to gender. If parents and children were in the same workhouse they were allowed a daily 'interview', although policy for each workhouse was at the discretion of the local board of guardians.

The harsh regimes and lax accountability of staff provided a potential environment for abuse. Workhouse schools – labelled 'Barrack schools' by their detractors – grew in size in the course of the nineteenth century, and this growth also provided conditions for institutional abuse. The Poor Law commissioners issued guidelines on corporal punishment: No female child was to be subject to corporal punishment nor could boys over 14 years of age be flogged. Boys under that age could only be punished by the master or schoolmaster (both had to be present) using a rod or other instrument specifically approved by the guardians. Despite the guidelines there were well publicized scandals throughout the nineteenth century in which children were found to be flogged severely. Other forms of exploitation remained more hidden such as the apprenticing of workhouse boys to individual members of the boards of guardians as a form of indentured labour.

Charlie Chaplin remembers

Charlie Chaplin (1889–1977) was just 7 years old when he, his brother and his mother, who suffered from mental health problems, entered the Lambeth Workhouse in 1896. He never forgot the experience, as he wrote in his autobiography:

> Although we were aware of the shame of going to the workhouse, when Mother told us about it both Sydney [his brother] and I thought it adventurous and a change from living in one stuffy room. But on that doleful day I didn't realize what was happening until we actually entered

the workhouse gate. Then the forlorn bewilderment of it struck me; for there we were made to separate, Mother going in one direction to the women's ward and we in another to the children's.

How well I remember the poignant sadness of that first visiting day: the shock of seeing Mother enter the visiting-room garbed in workhouse clothes. How forlorn and embarrassed she looked! In one week she had aged and grown thin, but her face lit up when she saw us.

(Chaplin 1964: 26)

The routes that children might take into the workhouse were at least three. First, if an able-bodied father entered the workhouse the entire family had to accompany him. Second, virtually from the start of the system, and certainly by the 1840s, workhouses were seen as care of the last resort for pauper orphans who had no other form of support. Indeed, boards of guardians were empowered to detain an orphan under the age of 16 if they thought the child would come to harm should they leave. Third, as concern developed regarding child neglect and physical cruelty to children, guardians were empowered to remove a child to the workhouse if the parents proved unfit – whether through alcoholism, mental deficiency or convicted of an offence against the child.

Child neglect in Leeds, 1861

The following report appeared in the *Leeds Mercury* of 14 March 1861 concerning a hearing at the police court in Leeds town hall.

Sarah Robinson, residing in Barrack street, Buslingthorpe Lane with her husband, Alfred Robinson (recently dismissed from the Leeds police force for drunkenness) was charged with having neglected and ill-treated her children. It was stated by Mr. English, the chief constable, that on the previous morning he received information that the defendant and her husband were in the habit of ill-treating and starving their children, and that they had actually rubbed the face of one of them with its own excrement. The children had also been so constantly deprived of food that they had gone to the neighbours' swill tubs and eaten the contents to satisfy their hunger. One of the children had been removed to the workhouse; the other, a boy about seven years of age, of very emaciated appearance, and whose back was covered with bruises, was present in court.

Mr. Chorely, magistrate, stated that he saw the child on Monday, and they were then in a very deplorable condition and evidently starving. He directed one of them to be removed to the workhouse, and that proceedings should be taken against the parents. The case was remanded until yesterday for the production of evidence, and both the husband and wife were then charged with the offence.

'Boarding out' under the Poor Law

The last thirty years of the nineteenth century saw increased effort to place children with foster parents outside the workhouse, or 'boarding out'. (As a term for fostering it survived late into the twentieth century long after the workhouses had closed.) Poor Law Amendment Acts in 1889 and 1899 gave guardians the right to assume parental rights and responsibilities over a child in their care until he or she was 18 – a significant development in the legal authority of the state over individual children, giving the state formal powers to foster children from the workhouse. While the law applied first to deserted children it was soon extended to include orphans, and children whose parents were disabled or unfit to have control over them. Parents had the right of appeal to a magistrates court but their chances were not strong: in 1908 alone some 12,400 children had their parental rights assumed by boards of guardians (Keating 2008: 25).

The move to board out began largely in rural areas in which children were placed with rural families ('cottagers') with small grants for food and clothing provided by the boards of guardians. Scotland, where boarding out had been informally practised all along, also pioneered the fostering of working-class children from urban workhouses by placing them with families in neighbouring rural districts where small farmers and crofters had the room and self-sustaining food sources to provide for two or more children. Learning from the Scottish model, English boards of guardians were permitted to board out children in districts other than their own from approximately 1870, but the system was used only sparingly at first and mostly for orphans, 'illegitimate' children abandoned by their mothers or children abandoned by both parents (Heywood 1978: 80). Concerns about the foster parents' receiving children for the maintenance allowance that came with them, as well as the foster parents' potential casual attitude towards the child's education, prompted a set of guidelines that, to one degree or another, have appeared regularly in social worker's duties towards fostered children (see box).

Regulations covering the boarding out of children within the Poor Law in 1870

Each board of guardians had to establish a boarding-out committee and each boarded out child had to be visited every six weeks by a member of the committee who must then report in writing on the child's condition. No child under 2 years of age could be boarded out, and all children had to have a certificate of good health before placement. A child could not be boarded out with foster parents of a different religious creed. Nor could children be placed with relations or in a home where the father was employed in night-work. The boarding-out committee had to inspect home arrangements: 'Special attention should be paid to decent accommodations and the proper separation of the sexes in the sleeping rooms. No child should be boarded out in a house where [there is] an adult

lodger.' Particular attention should be paid to the schoolmaster's quarterly report on the child – if unfavourable for two quarters in a row the child should be
instantly withdrawn. All children were to be sent out in good ordinary clothing
avoiding anything resembling a workhouse uniform.

Source: Poor Law Board 1870.

What we would regard as clear social work functions, such as regular visiting, inspection of accommodation, matching of religious creed, and checking
on progress in school, emerged from the regulations described in the box
above. They were carried out by volunteers overseen by the relieving officer of
the workhouses, in ways that paralleled the supervisory and reporting functions of visiting committee members operating under the Mental Deficiency
Act 1913. In this instance, however, these early volunteer social workers did
so on behalf of the Poor Law system.

Boarding out was by no means a universal practice. By the end of the
first decade of the twentieth century there were still well over 22,000 children
within the workhouse system, compared with 8,600 who were boarded out.
The limits of the policy, as Heywood has pointed out, lay in the absence of
people to undertake careful assessment of foster parents and supervision once
the placement was under way. In sum, 'As a skill boarding out was an empirical,
chancy piece of work, and it was realized that more attention needed to be
given to it' (Heywood 1978: 90). Increasingly there were calls to free children
from the stigma of the Poor Law altogether by placing boarding out in the
hands of competent women officers directly under the supervision of the Local
Government Board. Among the voices calling for this change were those of
the majority of the Royal Commission on the Poor Law that reported in 1909.

Emmeline Pankhurst remembers

Emmeline Pankhurst (1858–1928), a leading suffragette, was elected to the
board of guardians in Manchester in 1894. Years later, in her autobiography
My Own Story, she recounted her visits to children in the workhouses under her
responsibility.

> The first time I went into the place I was horrified to see little girls seven and
> eight years on their knees scrubbing the cold stones of the long corridors.
> These little girls were clad, summer and winter, in thin cotton frocks, low
> in the neck and short sleeved. At night they wore nothing at all, night
> dresses being considered too good for paupers. The fact that bronchitis was
> epidemic among them most of the time had not suggested to the guardians
> any change in the fashion of their clothes.

> I also found pregnant women in the workhouse, scrubbing floors, doing the hardest kind of work, almost until their babies came into the world. Many of them were unmarried women, very, very young, mere girls. These poor mothers were allowed to stay in the hospital after confinement for a short two weeks. Then they had to make a choice of staying in the workhouse and earning their living by scrubbing and other work, in which case they were separated from their babies. They could stay and be paupers, or they could leave – leave with a two-week-old baby in their arms, without hope, without home, without money, without anywhere to go. What became of those girls, and what became of their hapless infants?
>
> (Pankhurst 1914: 25)

School care committees

The introduction of compulsory primary education in 1880 revealed the extent of neglect and malnourishment among working-class children. Schools, especially the new 'Board schools' built in areas that previously had no school, provided ready data on the lives of children attending schools across the country. Soon after the formation of the London County Council (LCC) in 1889 its education committee noted that some 44,000 children were 'habitually underfed' – some 13 per cent of children attending school; not only were they 'semi-starved' but 'filthily dirty, sickly looking, with sore eyes and unwholesome aspect' (quoted in Willmott 2004: 2). A later LCC report noted several causes of child neglect including alcohol abuse, desertion by the father, unemployment, casual labour and low wages (Frere 1909).

The response in London and in some other local authorities was to call for the setting up of voluntary care committees across the different education authorities from which 'careful, regular and sympathetic home visiting' could be provided. These began their work in 1908; by 1929 there were an estimated five thousand volunteers working for them (Jennings 1930). Invariably the organizers of these committees were paid by the local authority; along with the COS family workers and the child protection officers of the NSPCC they were an early version of children's social workers. The Younghusband Report of 1959 (see Chapter 7) expressly noted that in the era before the Second World War, when there were few trained social workers employed by local authorities, among the earliest were the paid organizers of the care committees.

The role of the volunteer was to:

- undertake needs assessments for neglected, maladjusted or delicate children;
- be present at school medical examinations of specific children and to make follow-up visits to the family to explain the conclusions;

- oversee applications for clothing grants or for financial help for a school trip;
- decide whether specific pupils needed to attend a special school. (Frere 1909)

It is clear that both the organizers of the care committees and the volunteers identified their work as social work (Willmott 2004). They were women from upper professional and affluent backgrounds willing to devote a portion of their lives to the service of others. From the testimony that Willmott gathered from some of these volunteers you sense their shock in their first home visits. Problems that became all too familiar to a later generation of fieldworkers – no food in the house, obvious remains of enuresis and encopresis, children as young carers, overcrowding, cold and damp environments, mothers too ill to look after children, absent fathers – hit them hard in their first encounters with impoverished working-class life. They also learned that parents could resent the offer of assistance if linked to requests for further information about the family. As one parent said to a volunteer: 'The Council don't half want to know a lot for a bit of dinner, don't they?' (Jennings 1930).

Voluntary organizations and child rescue

Running in parallel with the Poor Law system for the care of orphaned, deserted children or those with 'unfit' parents, was a large but uncoordinated sector of voluntary charities also dedicated to child welfare. The period from the last third of the nineteenth century to the outbreak of the First World War saw an explosion in the number of organizations forming in response to abandoned, orphaned or homeless children of the urban working class. Child rescue work sprang from the same religious and evangelical soil as the temperance campaigns, campaigns against prostitution and animal cruelty. Dr Barnardo's (1867 – evangelical Irish Protestant), Waifs and Strays (1881 – Anglican, later the Children's Society), National Children's Homes (1870 – Methodist), Norwood Orphanage (1877 – Jewish) and Father Hudson Society (1902 – Catholic), all shared elements of the child rescue mission.[1] Most were founded by vigorous social entrepreneurs with a capacity for organization, prodigious work and a flair for self-publicity.[2] All were formed after their founders were moved by seeing numbers of children sleeping rough in the East End of London or other cities such as Birmingham. All offered homes for children but in time added further dimensions to their rescue work, developing fostering and adoption services as well as setting up arrangements for their children to emigrate to Canada, the United States or Australia. While their ethos reflected their founders' strong religious motivation, all proved remarkably durable, modernizing that ethos and reconstructing their services as required; all are in existence today.

George Stephenson and the founding of the National Children's Home

---

The Methodist minister George Stephenson and two colleagues converted an old stable block near Stephenson's chapel in the vicinity of Waterloo station in London. The aim was 'to rescue children, who through the death or vice or extreme poverty of their parents, are in danger of falling into criminal ways' (quoted in Philpot 1994: 23).

From the beginning, Stephenson wanted to avoid reproducing a new institution – he despaired of environments where large numbers of boys were housed together – and aimed to create a family atmosphere with small numbers of children looked after by house parents who were 'to encourage the boys to treat them with the respect, confidence and affection due to parents' (ibid.: 24). Although Stephenson spoke on occasion in missionary terms, he placed less emphasis on the need to save the souls of the young people, and the home itself was non-sectarian. Nevertheless a Christian spirit was to run through life in the home, with daily prayers and attendance at chapel twice on Sundays (ibid.).

The flow of children into the voluntary children's homes soon moved beyond rescue directly from the streets and came through diverse networks, including parents' own referrals, Poor Law guardians, and the NSPCC which ran no long-term homes of its own.

Alongside these national organizations were the efforts of local voluntary organizations which experimented with smaller residential homes for children based on clusters of cottages or single dwellings that adopted a family-group ethos as a way of teaching moral behaviour and self-responsibility under the tutelage of parent-like figures. In the years before the First World War these homes showed from our twenty-first-century perspective, a range of unregulated activity and hasty judgement glossed over with tales of happy endings.

The 'child rescue' model, at its extreme, was dependent on removal of a child from their current circumstances without much investigation into what those circumstances were, especially the relationship between parents and child and whether the parents wished the child to be rescued. There was little consideration of parental capacity or assessment of children's needs. The child's neighbourhood environment itself was regarded as the source of depravity from which the child had to be removed. Thomas Barnardo, for instance, thought the work generally to be a race against time – the children of the slums should be removed from their surroundings early enough and be kept sufficiently long to undertake training. As he put it: 'heredity counts for little, environment counts for everything' (quoted in Behlmer 1998: 291). Barnardo was zealous in his rescue of children and went so far as to confess that he had kidnapped a child in the 1880s.

On the other hand, the voluntary organizations, large and small, were conscious that it was necessary to find ways of looking after children, who could not be or were not looked after by their parents, outside the workhouse and the Poor Law system. With all its limitations – the lack of sensitivity to parental wishes and feelings, and particularly the egregious policy of sending children abroad for ever – the movement provided a stepping stone of sorts to more child-centred ways in looking after children.

Child protection

Victorian reformers were aware of certain aspects of the violence done to young children. In particular, 'baby farming' – the practice of receiving infants to nurse or rear in exchange for payment – was associated with criminality. The practice offered a version of child-minding for mothers going to work. At its worst it preyed on unmarried mothers and those with unwanted infants and produced a chain of scandals in which children were brought to near starvation or murdered outright through overdoses of narcotics or plain poison.

But tackling the problem of baby farming proved immensely difficult, a combination of the secrecy and the lack of evidence surrounding a practice shrouded in obscurity, a wariness about prying to closely into family affairs and the lack of a suitable agency to investigate and prosecute. Legislation regularly attempted to breakdown the factors that screened infanticide from the public eye: setting fines, for example, for failure to register a birth or neglecting to report finding an abandoned child. Other statutes prohibited graveyard officials from burying stillborn infants without a medical certificate stating that the child had been born dead. Giving a false statement or certificate could bring two years' imprisonment. But a legislative attempt in the early 1870s to allow the courts to appoint a guardian for a child under 12 whose parent had been convicted of bodily harm was never even debated in Parliament: the power given to the guardian to remove the child from the parent's custody if necessary was considered too intrusive.

The National Society for the Prevention of Cruelty to Children

Ten years later, in the 1880s, public mood regarding child abuse had changed. Concern grew not just over infanticide but over the practices of neglectful families and the need to ensure that working-class children were raised as responsible citizens. In 1883 a new voluntary agency to safeguard children was created, first in Liverpool (the Liverpool Society for the Prevention of Cruelty to Children) and then in London (the Society for the Prevention of Cruelty to Children, SPCC) the following year. Within a few years they merged, with other societies such as those in Edinburgh and Glasgow, to form the National Society for the Prevention of Cruelty to Children (NSPCC). The organizations arose from a well tested model of Victorian voluntary activity: letters in the local newspapers called for action prompting the formation of a coalition of local officials, magistrates, elected members of the boards of education, and leaders of the voluntary movement. The nationally respected Royal Society for the Prevention of Cruelty to Animals (RSPCA) provided direct assistance and advice to the new society – a link which it made much of in publicity. The local committees endeavoured to be inclusive, with members carefully drawn from different faiths – Anglican, Catholic and Nonconformist – and men and women.

The societies sought not only to tackle specific aspects of child abuse (the London Society in its first year campaigned vigorously for the criminalization of child sexual abuse) but also to bring moral guidance to parental conduct. Behind this lay what they saw as the need to discipline the chaotic family life of the urban lower working class – 'the residuum'.

There remained a wide gulf between what the NSPCC wanted to achieve and what the law said its officers were allowed to do in terms of investigation of alleged child abuse. The Prevention of Cruelty to, and protection of, Children Act 1889 was the first attempt in English law to deal with the domestic relationship between parent and child and to bring the law into line with the moral aims of child rescue. The NSPCC had lobbied hard for its main provisions, which it had largely drafted; public opinion shifting quickly towards reform was another pressure on Parliament.

The Act specified new offences in relation to children, defined as boys under 14 and girls under 16, and faithfully reflected the NSPCC's definition of child abuse:

- Neglect, ill treatment and abandonment were now punishable by a fine of £100 (double that if the accused were in some way making money out of the child's treatment) and up to two years' imprisonment, with or without hard labour.
- The procuring of children for hawking, begging and other forms of exploitation such as performing on licensed premises became a criminal offence.

The Act further introduced new tools which, in one format or another, survived for nearly one hundred years:

- It empowered a court to issue a warrant for any person to enter premises to search for a child, if that child was likely to be suffering unnecessarily, and to take the child to a 'place of safety'.
- The Act also empowered courts to give custody of a child to a relation or other 'fit person' – which included industrial schools or children's home – should it be necessary.

The Act maintained the popular view that momentous social effort could and should be shouldered exclusively by the voluntary sector. With regard to child abuse this consisted solely of the NSPCC. It had some thirty-five local committees but only a small number of inspectors to hand: two in its early years in London and no more than thirty nationally in the wake of the passage of the 1889 Act. From the start they were under pressure to meet the demands forged by the new legislation and the change in public attitudes.

While useful for purposes of publicity, the percentage of cases that came to the Society's attention involving outright cruelty to children diminished over time: from some 45 per cent in 1889 to just under 8 per cent before the First World War (Behlmer 1998). Behlmer argues that it was far easier for the Society to hold working-class parents to account, criticizing their lack of responsibility, than to examine the deeper roots of child neglect. The causes of parental abuse, as the Society saw it, arose from what the parents themselves had suffered earlier in their lives. Although the majority of its cases were working-class households, with alcohol dependency strongly indicated, NSPCC leaders argued that abuse was the habit of mind rather than related to low income. The NSPCC, like the COS, also opposed the introduction of free school meals, believing that properly applied persuasion would convince parents to feed their children and was preferable to the introduction of a national scheme to provide meals based on schools.

Equally delicate was the role of the NSPCC official – the 'cruelty man' – within the working-class family. Accusations of high-handedness, the occasions when neighbours would report a family and the balance of power between husband and wife and children all had to be negotiated. So too did the Society's determination to ensure that every child was vaccinated – bringing parents regularly to court for failure to do so.

The Society's inspectors achieved a degree of professionalism and job security rarely found within the voluntary sector. They tended to be middle-aged men with an earlier career (nearly half were former policemen), were paid and held a post for nearly eight years on average. They were trained in gathering information from the family, helped men to find work and arranged the placement of abused children through boards of guardians. Each inspector's decision – to dismiss a case, issue a warning or take a parent to court – was supervised by the branch secretary. In addition, the national organization sent personnel from London unannounced to examine case reports and the reliability of information gathered on specific families. This level of organization and professionalism, Behlmer concluded, surpassed that of the local authorities at the time (Behlmer 1982).

The Children Act 1908 consolidated earlier child protection legislation and instituted significant reforms relating to young offenders in court. It added a new offence of 'wilful cruelty', which included the failure to provide adequate food, clothing, medical aid or lodging and allowed courts to remove children from mothers who were prostitutes and dissolute parents. The legislation reflected the continuing broad strategy of the NSPCC towards making working-class parents responsible for their children, specifically singling out forms of negligence thought to be widespread in working-class families – 'overlaying' (suffocating the child inadvertently when sleeping in a shared bed) and scalding. It also required registration of foster homes with only one child, where the foster parents received payment – previously only homes with two or more foster children had to register.

The Children Act 1908

The Act provided that 'any person' could bring before the court a child who was:

- found begging, wandering and not having any home or settled abode;
- found destitute with parents in prison;
- under the care of a parent or guardian unfit to have care of the child by reason of 'criminal or drunken habits';
- the daughter of a man convicted of sexual offences;
- living in a place of prostitution.

The court – now a juvenile court established for the first time by the Act – was to enquire into the matter and, if satisfied that one of the above conditions held, could commit the child to the care of a 'fit person'.

From the NSPCC records: Anne Purcell, 13$\frac{1}{2}$, of York, talks to the NSPCC in 1898

'Last night about 5.30 pm father came home. I took baby off the couch and my father saw it had dirtied on it. He took a towel and hit me with it, and when I put baby in the chair, he took off his strap and beat me as hard as he could over my arm and back with the buckle end of it – I did not scream out – I dare not for he would have hit me more. He hit me three or four times. My arm hurts me now, and nursing the baby makes it worse.

'After you and the policeman had left this dinnertime, my father asked me who I had told about him beating me – I said "The neighbours" – He then put his fist in my face and said – "If you go out this afternoon I'll cut you in two." He swore at me and said "You are going away you little B——, and a B——y good job."'

The NSPCC inspector wrote to the Secretary of the York branch:

'The child is exceedingly short for her age, and so bow-legged to be almost a cripple. To see and hear this child, and to note her anxiety as to the consequences to herself of anything she tells against her father, is most distressing to the onlooker. I sincerely hope something may be done for her.'

The father, George Purcell was prosecuted for assault on his daughter and was sent to prison for two months. A follow up visit six months after his release indicated that he had completely reformed and 'that Anne was a good housekeeper to him'.

Source: Case file in Behlmer 1982: 235–6.

The changing legal framework: adoption

Up to the end of the First World War the distinction between 'fostering' and 'adoption' was blurred. The state-sanctioned system for boarding out of children from workhouses, discussed above, sat side by side with a range of private and voluntary activity which placed children with families for longer or shorter durations and under varying conditions with families. From our perspective in which adoption is meticulously planned and investigated it comes as a shock to realize that, until the 1920s, adoption of children by adults who were not their parents was purely by informal arrangement in which neither courts nor the state had any part to play. Indeed, the terms 'adoption' and 'boarding out' were often used interchangeably until after the First World War, not least by boards of guardians themselves.

Mrs Waters' advertisement

Margaret Waters ran a classic baby farm in the 1870s. Five infants died in her care; she was found guilty of murder and executed. For weeks she had run the following advertisement in her local paper:

Adoption – A good home, with a mother's love and care, is offered to any respectable person wishing her child to be entirely adopted. Premium £5, which sum includes everything.

(quoted in Keating 2008: 23)

Voluntary adoption societies, however, began to match children with adoptive parents more carefully. The National Children's Home mentioned above fostered younger children with 'approved families', and although the children usually returned to the children's home, some were adopted by their foster parents in this de facto sense – some 260 by 1920. In 1920 the Salvation Army also reported some 500 adoptions over the previous thirty years.

Pressure to place adoption on a statutory basis increased dramatically in the aftermath of the First World War. War produced a range of social consequences that could not be ignored – war widows who could not look after their children, war orphans, the rise in the number of 'illegitimate children' born to unmarried mothers – impinged on the public consciousness. Informal fostering and putting infants out 'to nurse' was less an option as women had found higher wages in war-related industries. After the war, two major organizations – the National Children Adoption Association (NCAA) and the National Adoption Society (NAS) – engaged in what it called 'complete adoption'. Both accepted only healthy babies; both ran hostels for babies awaiting adoption; and both relied on secrecy in adoption practice: natural parents were never told where the new child's home was, unless expressly agreed to by the adopting parents. Parents giving up the child would sign a document stating that they were giving up their child but were also informed that there was no law that made this binding. There were some differences too: the NCAA made it clear that it would arrange adoption for children of all backgrounds – orphan, illegitimate or abused child, whereas the NAS placed a child with its new family on trial for a month, after which the child could be returned.

Led by the NAS and NCAA all the major children's voluntaries and diocesan associations involved in adoption campaigned to place adoption on a legal footing in the early 1920s (Keating 2001). Their chief aim was to ensure that adoptive parents would be secure in a legal entitlement to the child that natural parents could not overturn. The welfare of the child was not prominent in these discussions, with the general view prevailing that adopted children should be prepared to take what comes.

It is clear that as the debate unfolded the major adoption societies pressed for a particular kind of adoption process, one based on anonymity and the fear that natural parents would interfere and disrupt the process. There were countervailing voices. The Maternal and Child Welfare division of the Ministry of Health regarded the behaviour of adoption societies as focused solely on 'wholesale adoption' when it was preferable to keep mother and baby together. Its head, Zoe Puxley, raised the possibility of providing mothers with a pension or allowance as a way of offsetting the need for adoption. Others also argued for a state subsidy of unmarried mothers, although early campaigners for a family allowance, including Elizabeth Rathbone, rejected the idea.

Adoption Act 1926

The Adoption Act 1926 for the first time provided for a court order that transferred all rights, duties, obligations and liabilities for a child to the adopting parents, an order that was irrevocable. For this to happen, the child's parents had to understand that the order was irrevocable; their consent was required unless the court had dispensed with that consent. Significantly, the Act did *not* include the principle announced in the Guardianship Act of the year before, that the welfare of the child should be the paramount consideration before the court when determining guardianship; but it did acknowledge that the order should be for the welfare of the child and take into consideration the wishes of the child having regard to the age and understanding of the child.

The Act heralded the evolution of adoption from essentially a private transaction based on a contractual agreement between two parties to a process largely administered by social work agencies in the years ahead. In 1926 that process was just beginning. Adoption, while put on a legal footing, was not yet regulated by the state in any way and a freewheeling practice still existed around placement. A proliferation of voluntary adoption societies, tasteless advertisements claiming to come from children wanting to be adopted, a sometimes overly casual approach to vetting would-be adopters, the exchange of money, and sending babies abroad were all part of the process moving into the 1930s.

By the late 1930s the Home Office was aware of the shortcomings and called together a departmental committee with Florence Horsburgh MP as chair. The committee's recommendations were reflected in the Adoption of Children (Regulation) Act 1939 – one of the most important prewar markers in shifting the balance of social work activity from voluntary to state activity. The Act and ensuing regulations stipulated that no society should be allowed to arrange adoptions unless it was registered with the local authority, under regulations set by the Home Secretary governing placement procedures. It also sought to reduce significantly the number of adoptions still taking place between individuals by requiring prospective adopters to apply to court for an adoption order – although it did not recommend that private adoptions should end altogether.

Work with juvenile offenders

The distinction between criminal behaviour and behaviour of troubled children hardened by poverty was constantly debated, as in our own time.

'Hooliganism' (as anti-social behaviour was then called), the value of 'short, sharp shocks', the degree of leniency shown and the extent and expense of re-habilitative programmes were all issues regularly revisited in the discussion and politics surrounding youth crime. No single solution to the issue of juve-nile crime made significant impact. One alternative was the privately run reformatory school to which young offenders could be sent after a short period in prison. Industrial schools run by various voluntary organizations with grants from the state were also developed largely providing for younger children in which both offenders and those on the brink of crime could find an approximation of parental-like supervision and correction missing in their own homes. They, too, were found to have their limitations as their regimes tended to be similar to reformatories and as parents were deemed by magistrates to be deliberately citing 'loss of control' of their young per-son in the hope that the state would give them residence and training at its expense.

The emergence of a social work function in relation to juvenile offenders began with the Church of England Temperance Society providing volunteers willing to offer guidance to offenders in magistrates courts from the mid-1870s. By 1900 this service had developed into 'prison gate missions', meeting those freshly released from prison with guidance and support for those who wanted it. The Anglican roots of probation lie in these police court missionaries and reassured lawmakers and magistrates that the notion of a national probation service would introduce the right kind of balance between moral uplift and upholding the law in their work with young offenders. One of the first juvenile courts in the country – Birmingham – took on three full-time children's officers in 1906. In 1907 a voluntary probation service was established, while the Children Act 1908 introduced a system of juvenile courts for offenders under 16. In the same year the system of Borstal training (named after the village in Kent where a prototype establishment was sited), was established for offenders aged between 16 and 21.

Juvenile crime increased substantially and suddenly during the First World War but fell away again as quickly once war was over. In the 1920s nearly one-fifth of juvenile offenders coming before the courts were placed on probation – yet there were still courts without a probation officer. Nor was the practice of juvenile courts standardized and it was still a rare occasion for a young of-fender to find magistrates with informed insight into child behaviour or a courtroom with an informal atmosphere (Bailey 1987: 41). There was argu-ment also over the nature of the probation service and whether it should remain in the hands of voluntary organizations – principally the Church of England Temperance Society – or whether probation officers should be or-ganized and paid by the state. Leading voices such as William Clarke Hall (see below) and Margery Fry of the Howard League for Penal Reform (an or-ganization with nineteenth-century roots) argued for the latter while other critics also argued that the link between the Church of England police court missionaries and the church's temperance movement should be separated; they were supported by those who argued that social work in Britain was traditionally carried out by voluntary organizations and this should apply to probation work.

As so often in the evolution of social work, a compromise of sorts was worked out in the Criminal Justice Act 1925 that effectively established a national probation service based on 'dual control' under state and voluntary organizations.

- Each area was to have an appointed, paid probation officer overseen by a probation committee of magistrates, with the cost shared between the Treasury and the local authority. Local magistrates were left free to choose between appointing agents from the voluntary societies or their own officers to carry out probation work.
- The voluntary Church of England Temperance Society was guaranteed official standing; it continued to make a significant financial contribution to the service as well as retain denominational tests on many probation officers.
- The Conservative government of the time directly urged magistrates to select probation officers 'because they want to rescue the perishing, because they want to raise up the fallen, because they want to take a human soul and bring it back to God' (quoted in Bailey 1987: 44).

Social conception of delinquency

The Children's Branch of the Home Office was intent on promoting a youth justice practice based on what can be called a 'social conception of delinquency' that lay at the heart of work with young offenders in the 1920s and 1930s. One of its exponents was William Clarke Hall (1866–1932), a former president of Toynbee Hall and prosecuting counsel for the NSPCC, who knew the children and families of the East End of London. In his practice as a magistrate in the juvenile court and in a series of publications he argued that juvenile courts should examine the causes of a child's delinquency and reach an informed decision as to a preventive response. Another advocate, Cyril Burt, had become interested in delinquency from his time in residence in a university settlement in Liverpool. As psychologist to the education department of the London County Council, Burt examined the impact of poverty, poor schooling and unemployment on delinquency. Ultimately he argued that 'inner personal weakness' made individual young people susceptible to delinquency rather than drawing a straight causal link with poor environment, but he did argue that delinquency was 'dangerous perhaps and extreme, but none the less typical – of common childish naughtiness' (Burt 1925: viii).

The debate on the causes of youth crime and influences on young offenders was thus joined and has remained with us to this day, best summarized between what are loosely called the justice model and the welfare model of youth offending. Should young offenders be treated as 'children in need' or as criminals deserving punishment? If the former, what kind of 'preventive work' or 'treatment' is required to neutralize their environment? If the latter, what penal regime is appropriate?

The changing legal framework: the role of the local authority

In the 1920s and 1930s social work continued to be performed across a matrix of different sectors and functions. Nowhere was this more evident than in child welfare:

- Care committees continued to be organized by the local authority under the auspices of its education committee. The committee organizers were paid but they relied wholly on volunteers for the family visiting and support.
- Work with unsupported mothers was undertaken by faith-based moral welfare workers – increasingly working in partnership with the local authority.
- Child protection work was undertaken by a single prominent voluntary organization, well known in working-class neighbourhoods, the NSPCC.
- School attendance officers employed by the local authority ensured just that – they had not yet become education welfare officers of the postwar era.
- Psychiatric social workers worked with children with behavioural difficulties through independent child guidance clinics.
- Probation officers dealt with troublesome and delinquent teenagers.

As diverse as voluntary services for children were, when it came to the major concerns around child neglect and cruelty, governmental authority was the ultimate authority: it alone had the capacity and the national impact to implement a coordinated strategy. Boards of guardians were finally abolished by the Local Government Act 1929, with the central administration of poor relief for children given to the Ministry of Health. This included the care of orphans and neglected children. At the same time, local authorities became responsible for the day-to-day running of poor relief, including children in need, acting through newly established Public Assistance Committees which the 1929 Act obliged them to set up. Thus were local authorities directly brought into the oversight of children's services even if in areas of moral welfare, mental deficiency and child protection they continued to rely on provisions from the voluntary sector.

The Children and Young Persons Act 1933 – and similar legislation in Scotland in 1937 – made the local authority primarily responsible for bringing children in need of care and protection before the court, a duty which under the 1908 Children Act had rested with the police.[3] The power to initiate proceedings was now restricted to the local authority, the police and the NSPCC. It also made the local authority responsible for those children subject of a 'fit person order'. In general, local authorities discharged their new responsibility through their education departments which were empowered by the Act to place children committed to their care into foster homes. Local authorities also took on increased responsibility for residential and foster care.

The 1933 Act enshrined the social conception of delinquency in law – making no distinction between the treatment of a young offender and providing for a young person in need. The philosophy behind the Act saw the young offender's environment as the source of his delinquency. The Home Office circular that accompanied the Act noted that there was little difference in the character of the child as offender or as victim of cruelty or neglect and the methods for dealing with each child were similar (Home Office 1933: 2). The Act directed any court dealing with a child or young person – whether an offender or in need of care and protection – to have regard for the welfare of that child, and in so doing finally gave the notion of the child's welfare legal standing although it was not yet paramount.

*   *   *   *

Between approximately 1870 and 1939 important markers were laid down in statute and in practice pointing towards greater state involvement in the lives of disadvantaged or neglected children. The capacity of the state to remove a child from unfit parents was established, as was the state's power to regulate adoption activities. The position of the NSPCC remained pre-eminent in dealing with child abuse, but the first steps were already established through which the local authority would eventually, after a second momentous world war, take a lead role in that area of work as well.

	PUBLIC SECTOR	VOLUNTARY SECTOR
PAID	Relieving officers (from 1930 Area Welfare Officers) -overseeing boarding out from work house up to 1909	NSPCC agents
		CAMW officers
		COS District officers
		Settlement house workers
	Care committee organizers	Adoption society staff
	Probation Officers (under Home Office after 1926)	'Bible women'
		Anglican temperance missionaries as probation officers (1876-1926)
		PSWs in child guidance clinics
		Moral welfare agency staff
UNPAID	Care committee volunteer visitors	Children's visiting societies' volunteers to work-house, child-minded, & boarded out children
	Infant Life Protection visitors	Adoption society visitors
	Boarded out children's visitors	Moral welfare visitors with unmarried mothers (Anglican, Methodist, Catholic, Jewish)
		COS family visitors

Figure 6.1 Children's social work services on eve of Second World War

Summary

- Children's services were slowly and only partially detached from the operation of the Poor Law.
- The Poor Law authorities themselves undertook a practice of 'boarding out' children from the workhouse.
- The voluntary sector engaged in 'child rescue', sometimes with little systematic appraisal of a child's needs or their parents' capacities.
- Cruelty to children was eventually recognized as a distinct social problem in the 1870s and 1880s; the first organization to deal with it on a national scale was the NSPCC.
- Adoption was not given a legal footing until 1926.
- Gender played a critical role in early social work: the volunteer school care committees were all women; the NSPCC inspectors were all male; boards of guardians were largely all male until the late nineteenth century when women were more widely appointed or elected.

Notes

1. The first three of these were the largest, accounting for nearly half of the voluntary effort in this field.
2. Thomas John Barnardo added 'Dr' as a title although he was not medically trained in any way. The title stuck, and indeed his organization was referred to as 'Dr Barnardo's' long after his death in 1903 at the age of 60. He would also have photographs of children retouched for the newspapers to make them visually more persuasive for the public.
3. Part of the 1933 Act – 'Schedule 1 offenders' convicted of rape, incest and abandonment – survived well into the late twentieth century.

Suggested reading

Bailey, V. (1987). *Delinquency and Citizenship: Reclaiming the Young Offender 1914–1948*. Oxford: Clarendon Press.

Behlmer, G. (1982). *Child Abuse and Moral Reform in England, 1870–1908*. Stanford, CA: Stanford University Press.

Heywood, J. (1978). *Children in Care: The Development of the Service for the Deprived Child*. London: Routledge & Kegan Paul.

Keating, J. (2008). *A Child for Keeps: The History of Adoption in England 1918–1945*. Basingstoke: Palgrave Macmillan.

Part Two
The Road to Modernization

SOCIAL WORK TIMELINE 1939–2010

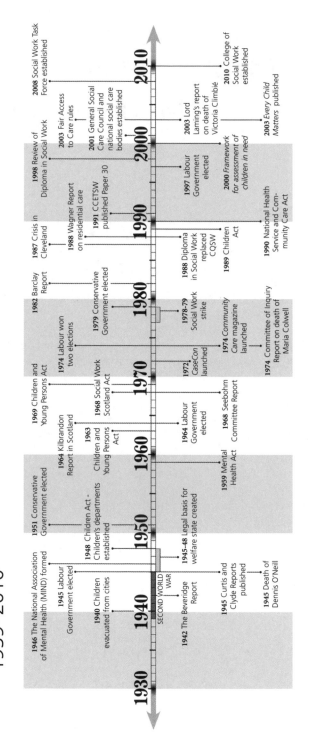

1930

1940

SECOND WORLD WAR

1950

1960

1970

1980

1990

2000

2010

1946 The National Association of Mental Health (MIND) formed

1945 Labour Government elected

1940 Children evacuated from cities

1951 Conservative Government elected

1948 Children's departments established

1945–48 Legal basis for welfare state created

1942 The Beveridge Report

1945 Curtis and Clyde Reports published

1945 Death of Dennis O'Neill

1964 Kilbrandon Report in Scotland

1963 Children and Young Persons Act

1959 Mental Health Act

1969 Children and Young Persons Act

1968 Social Work Scotland Act

1964 Labour Government elected

1968 Seebohm Committee Report

1974 Labour won two elections

1979 Conservative Government elected

1972 *CaseCon* launched

1974 *Community Care* magazine launched

1974 Committee of Inquiry Report on death of Maria Colwell

1982 Barclay Report

1978–79 Social Work strike

1987 Crisis in Cleveland

1988 Wagner Report on residential care

1991 CCETSW published Paper 30

1988 Diploma in Social Work replaced CQSW

1989 Children Act

1990 National Health Service and Community Care Act

1998 Review of Diploma in Social Work

1997 Labour Government elected

2000 *Framework for assessment of children in need*

2008 Social Work Task Force established

2003 Fair Access to Care rules

2001 General Social Care Council and national social care bodies established

2003 Lord Laming's report on death of Victoria Climbié

2010 College of Social Work established

2003 *Every Child Matters* published

7 Social Work At High Tide: From the Second World War to Single Social Services Department

This chapter covers the developments in social work from the Second World War to the setting up of the unified social services departments as recommended by the Seebohm Committee in 1968. It discusses:

- the impact of the war on social work;
- the dominance of casework as social work method;
- the work of the Seebohm Committee and the eventual establishment of single local authority social services departments;
- the unification of social work as a profession;
- the plurality of methods that emerged as social casework lost its influence.

The thirty years following the end of the Second World War in 1945 are often regarded as a time when politicians, the public and practitioners themselves looked upon social work as a selfless activity aiming to do good (White 2011). It was a period when the social work mission was as yet unsullied by publicly derided failure, when budgets and resources were increased regularly, and confidence of practitioners in their mission was high. When an older generation of social workers refers to a golden era, this is the time they look back to. Unity is the central theme of this chapter – unifying social work services in a single local authority department, unifying the myriad professional associations into a single professional association and unifying social work method in social work education.

Social work and the welfare state

The 'people's war' mobilized the nation in a common cause against a mortal threat, and the entire population underwent common experiences. It exacted a high toll on civilian life and limb in the working-class and industrial districts of its major cities. Men were called up across the social classes; women entered the armed forces in unprecedented numbers; industrial production relied on a disciplined labour force and the cooperation of trade unions.

War demanded a high degree of organization on the home front in ways that foreshadowed approaches to social policy after the war. The Emergency Medical Service, for example, enforced coordination of health services and paid GPs' salaries. Food was rationed and coordinated in distribution. Supplementary pensions were paid to older people suffering hardship. The limitations of hospitals, maternity units, nurseries and welfare clinics were also ruthlessly exposed.

Above all the evacuation of children made substantial sections of public opinion and policy makers realize that 'the skinnies' – the under nourished working class children – were not the consequence of a few problem families but of poor nutrition endemic for those on low income (Holman 1995). Evacuation occurred in two waves: at the outset of war in 1939, before military engagement started, and then again in 1940 when the bombing campaigns began in earnest. The result was a culture shock on both sides. The foster parents who received evacuee children were largely middle class and based in rural areas or small towns; they found they had to wrestle with behaviour problems such as bed-wetting and problematic manners, and poor eating habits. For the children, evacuated from urban working-class families, both the experience and the environment were strange and new.

To smooth the settling-in process, local authorities responded by increasing the number of visitors from care committees to support and advise foster parents. Children showing disturbed behaviour were supported by psychiatric social workers – with referrals often coming from the volunteer visitors. Local authorities also created some 700 children's homes and hostels to receive those evacuated children whose behaviour was beyond that which a family could reasonably control. Some of these establishments were linked to psychiatric consultants such as Donald Winnicott in Oxfordshire who began to investigate the effects of group care on children (Holman 1995).

The national government elected in 1935 – mostly Conservative but with some National Liberals – evolved into a broad wartime coalition that included the Labour Party. A general election was deferred until the end of the war. The publication of the Beveridge Report (1942) promised that after the war Britain would create what only later came to be called a 'welfare state', in which basic needs were to be met largely through public provision – old age pension, family allowance, care in old age, unemployment insurance and a basic social security. The election of a Labour government in July 1945 was due in no small part to the Labour Party's unqualified support for the report's recommendations whereas the Conservatives held back on full endorsement. From a largely ad hoc system of welfare, localized, voluntary and small scale before the war, a public welfare system emerged that was relatively centralized.

Key legislation setting up the welfare state after 1945
1945   Family Allowance Act – introduced state-funded child benefit, following a thirty-year campaign by Elizabeth Rathbone and others. 1946   National Health Service Act (implemented in 1948) – nationalized the patchwork system of voluntary and former Poor Law and municipal hospitals and brought GPs, who remained self-employed, directly into the provision of health care free at the point of use. 1948   National Insurance Act – provided cover for sickness, unemployment, disability and retirement, replacing earlier schemes which largely covered only male workers. 1948   National Assistance Act – gave local authority welfare departments responsibilities for providing residential and other services for older people, the physically disabled and the homeless; this so-called Part III accommodation, after that part of the Act remained a fixture for social workers into the 1980s. 1948   Children Act – compelled local authorities to set up children's departments, under newly appointed children's officers, to handle public child care and social work with children.

Social work in late 1940s and 1950s

Social work found itself practising within a new social compact between state and citizen, one underpinned by a comprehensive system of income support for those who could not participate in the labour market and health care free at the point of use, a system quite different from the individualist, voluntary, local ethos of which previously it had been both a product and enthusiastic supporter. Social work had little difficulty in assimilating itself to this social democratic framework. As we noted in Part One, prewar attitudes towards state-provided services were already changing among the various ranks of the salaried personnel who undertook social work functions. Major voluntary organizations were also modernizing as they developed greater understanding of the complexities of human needs (see Figure 7.1).

Yet there was a broader question to answer: what was the role of social work to be when most needs were being met by a comprehensive welfare state? In response, social work came to see itself as the 'drop of oil' in the engine (McDougall and Cormack 1950: 30) – that is, given the universality

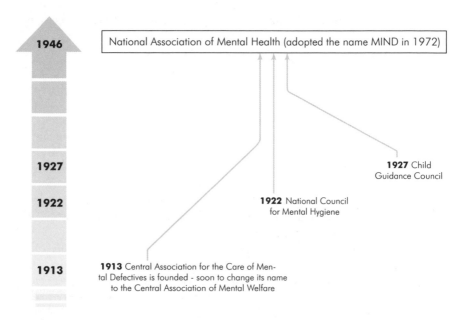

Figure 7.1 Voluntary organizations come of age: Formation of the National Association of Mental Health 1946. It emerged from a war time need when the Ministry of Health asked a coalition of mental health voluntary organizations to provide care for military personnel discharged from service on psychiatric grounds.

of income supports and other services that prewar practitioners could only dream about, social workers saw their work now as focusing on the needs of those individuals who could not or would not adapt themselves to the new welfare state.

Casework in mid-twentieth century

Casework was only part of what social workers actually did. Indeed, Eileen Younghusband in her first report on social work training after the Second World War had not used the term 'casework' in urging schools of social work to establish a wider curriculum for a range of workers (Younghusband 1947). Nevertheless, by 1950, 'casework', or 'social casework', had become virtually synonymous with social work: 'a distinctive orientation or approach to human problems, rather than a method or range of techniques' (Yelloly 1980: 97). 'The basis of all casework is the natural human response of one individual to another in some need,' as McDougall and Cormack (1950: 16) put it. While proponents were happy to place it side by side with other aspects of social work, such as collective action, group work and community work, casework was 'the natural human response' to 'natural human situations' (ibid.: 17), meeting a need which a person cannot meet unaided.

Casework theory was folded into the social democratic framework of the welfare state: while most people would have most of their essential needs met by universal provision, social work was required to provide detailed and comprehensive consideration of the troubled exceptions that can disrupt welfare systems completely. The Younghusband Committee looking into the role and function of social work heard that a local authority social worker should 'assess the disturbance of equilibrium in a given handicapped person and in his family and social relationships so as to give appropriate help' (Younghusband 1959: 174). Helping people in particular difficulties to adjust to an essentially benign society with guaranteed safety nets was a function that looked back to Mary Richmond and forward to the ideas of 'maintenance' in the 1980s as the prime objective. In the words of the Younghusband Report, social work looked to 'achieve the best possible personal, family and social adjustment' and should assume for the socially inadequate 'responsibilities beyond their [i.e. the families'] capacity to shoulder' (ibid.).

The fundamental basis of casework was the uniqueness of each individual, but there was also a presumption that clients were in a state of dependency. As a postwar definition put it: 'casework is the process of giving such attention and study to an individual and his environment as will enable him and the case-worker to work together, using all the resources available in the whole situation, to supply some need which is more than he could deal with by himself' (McDougall and Cormack 1950: 28). While acknowledging that people were social animals linked to their communities, the individual was the unit for which casework is responsible.

In terms of what social workers actually did, completing a 'social history' remained the vehicle through which the social worker amassed as much knowledge and information as possible: 'the history is really the picture which the case-worker makes of the client out of the information given by the client... out of the impression the client makes, and out of the resources of experience and theory which she has acquired in her training and in her work' (ibid.: 40). The history delved into all aspects of the client's past – what kind of child they were, and whether they were brought up to be independent or whether initiative was discouraged. School behaviour, ability to mix with others, work record were all subject to fact-finding in order to indicate the degree of willingness to shoulder the normal responsibilities of adult life. Assessments of personality were also routine – cheerful, moody, reserved, quarrelsome, lethargic. And following casework convention developed over thirty years, a diagnosis was reached, often through a conference between different agencies. 'Treatment' was largely made through interviews in which insight and changed attitudes were sought, built on the relationship with the case-worker.

At the time Father Biestek (1961), Helen Perlman (1957) and others provided a set of principles still adhered to today:

- Individuals are unique.
- Social workers should listen in an attentive, non-critical and non-directive way.
- The social worker's use of self is an important tool in building a relationship with a client.
- The client's right to self-determination should be respected.

These formulations of casework principles stemmed largely from contemporary American writing and were relatively new in Britain. According to Yelloly (1980: 97), British social workers, seeking to shake free from their long history of paternalist thinking, found the tenets forward looking. Although attacked by a later generation of radical social workers, both Craig Cawthorn (2010) and Tom White (2011) give testimony to the feeling of competence and worth that social casework theory gave practitioners.

Casework and psychoanalysis

If there is debate about how far social work in Britain before the war fell for the 'psychiatric deluge', there is no doubt that after the war psychodynamic casework, drawing on psychoanalysis, dominated the field. At this time psychoanalysis in Britain proved to be a remarkably fertile field, stimulated by the work of exceptional analyst-theorists based in London as they addressed the specific problems that wartime presented. Sigmund Freud himself was forced to flee Vienna in 1937 after the Nazis took power in Austria; he settled in London with his daughter Anna who had also trained in psychoanalysis and worked in children's nurseries in Hampstead during the war. Another continental refugee, Melanie Klein, and one of Klein's students, John Bowlby, applied some of the insights of psychoanalysis to understanding children's behaviour and needs in a practical way. Bowlby's work on attachment theory is the most familiar and enduring work from that period but there was impressive practice across several fields: Klein's own work on 'splitting' and encountering 'the other', the work of Anna Freud with children and Clare and Donald Winnicott's work with abandoned children collectively formed a distinctively British contribution to work with children (see Chapter 11). There were distinctive psychoanalytic contributors in other fields too. Wilfred Bion, a tank commander in the First World War and army psychiatrist in the Second, developed his influential dynamics of group work with soldiers suffering from what we now would recognize as post-traumatic stress syndrome. The work of other analysts with those with personality disorder provided further examples of direct engagement with social problems.

Sigmund Freud (1856–1939)

Freud, the celebrated founder of psychoanalysis, asserted he had discovered a new science of the personality based on several key points:

- Sexuality is important in childhood and its development can become arrested or distorted.
- Instinctual gratification is an important driver of human behaviour, particularly when constrained or thwarted by social custom and laws and needs to be harnessed for social and individual achievement.
- The 'Oedipus Complex' – the wish to 'marry' the parent of the opposite sex and to displace the rival parent.
- Fear of retribution for these Oedipal feelings are resolved by internalizing the parents' own authorities and commands becoming, in Freud's concept, the *superego* which can in fact extend beyond the parents to include objects of various disciplining authorities.

Freud noticed how some patients seemed to dwell on their suffering and regress at the point when treatment seemed promising – what he called 'the repetition-compulsion', the tendency to seek out and repeat traumatic experiences. In his later work Freud developed a wider concept of internal conflict – between the life instinct (which included sexuality) and a death instinct. On the basis of this he argued that the common wish for oblivion or death would be thwarted by society and turn outward in the form of aggression or elements of sadism – or inwards in masochism. Perhaps most importantly for casework theorists he uncovered what he called 'transference', that is, feelings and emotions drawn from other significant relationships of the patient are transferred to the analyst, and 'counter-transference' in which the analyst's emotions are focused on the patient. His methods of treatment were dream analysis, free association of the patient's thoughts and lengthy analytic sessions stretching over years in some cases.

In the postwar world, social work was strongly attracted to this orientation that seemed to unlock so many mysteries and at the same time was producing an innovative, distinctly British practice. Social workers accepted that they were not psychoanalysts and could not use its methods directly, but they could draw on some of the insights of psychoanalysis to inform their practice. Nor was this 'psychosocial' casework conceived as covert opposition to the new welfare state, but was seen instead as a product of it. John Bowlby's politics were emphatically social democratic and he viewed his work on attachment through that prism (see Chapter 10). Both Cawthorn (2010) and White (2010) explain how this psychodynamic vision of casework was empowering for social workers. It provided an orientation, a founding perspective, a way of looking at the world even if they adopted only small parts of it as their day-to-day method.

Barbara Wootton's critique of casework

Casework had its critics. The British sociologist Barbara Wootton (1897–1988) examined the major casework theorists such as Richmond, Younghusband and Hamilton, and found them fuzzy. She wrote:

> modern definitions of 'social casework', if taken at their face value, involve claims to powers which verge upon omniscience and omnipotence: one can only suppose that those who perpetuate these claims in cold print must, for some as yet unexplained reason, have been totally deserted by their sense of humour. Thus Mary Richmond, who is widely regarded as the founder of modern casework, once defined this as 'the art of doing different things for and with different people by co-operating with them to achieve at one and the same time their own and society's betterment' – a formula inclusive enough to cover any and every kind of altruistic activity.
>
> (Wootton 1959: 271)

Wootton argued that a caseworker could actually achieve those objectives more efficiently if she simply married her client (Wootton 1959).

Family Service Unit's broad definition of casework

Some practitioners, particularly in the voluntary sector, agreed with Wootton's critique. The Pacifist Service Units (PSUs) – set up initially to assist families struggling during the Second World War and shortly renamed Family Service Units (FSU) – developed a holistic approach that paid due attention to the material needs of the families but also offered intensive guidance and emotional support to achieve a stable family. In many ways the FSU anticipated community social work and work around social exclusion, particularly as it saw the complex inter-relationship between family behaviour and poverty. In a key pamphlet of 1945 it said:

> Often the attempt to find solutions for limited problems within the home results in the necessary break-up of the family especially in matters of child neglect, school attendance and delinquency. Symptoms of disintegration such as under-feeding, lack of discipline and dirty conditions, cannot be singled out from the general situation in the home and treated as if they were isolated problems. In dealing with such families it is therefore of the utmost importance for the caseworker to be in a position to treat every aspect of their distress.
>
> (Stephens 1945: 19)

Social casework and social work methods

By the 1960s casework as a method was coming under some pressure. It was resource-intensive, and difficult to evaluate. Already in the 1950s a version dubbed 'short contact interviewing' outlined how a productive relationship could be forged in a short time to accomplish casework tasks: develop a comprehensive picture, reach a quick diagnosis, and forward on to appropriate agency for help. This compression of casework accelerated in the 1960s, typified by *Brief and Extended Casework* (Reid and Shyne 1969) and subsequently the task-centred work (Reid and Epstein 1972) that emerged from it. This latter version was constructed around a maximum of eight encounters, gave greater voice to clients in defining problems to be tackled, and broke those problems down into small, achievable tasks agreed with the client. It also offered a way of documenting evidence in achieving social work aims and remains social work's only home-grown evidence-based method readily understood by clients. Other formulations, such as that by Eric Sainsbury (1970), a practising probation officer and lecturer at Sheffield University, deconstructed the familiar elements of casework, democratizing them, so to speak, and laying the groundwork for greater levels of user participation in the process.

By then reform was in the air – not just in relation to social work methods but also in the way services were to be delivered.

The Seebohm Committee and the single social services department

The debate in the mid-1960s about the future shape of social work took place at a time when public and politicians placed high value on social work. Since the war, various committees of enquiry concerned with services for groups of people with particular needs had regularly called for more social workers: to work with those with physical and learning disabilities, disabled children, those with chronic illness, delinquent youth, alcoholics and homeless families. As Cooper (1983) observed the reason for this was not that such calls were looking to social work professional expertise but that they recognized that the social systems of the welfare state needed mediators and advocates. She also noted that social workers had become adept through their various associations in publicising their skills, knowledge and roles in relation to particular client groups and that this strategy had produced a favourable public image.

As a result proposals to overcome the fragmentation of social work services became a high profile issue for government and social policy commentators alike with a number of different possibilities under debate. The Younghusband Report (1959) had called for greater coordination among social work services but not unification. David Donnison (Donnison et al. 1962), on the other hand, argued that a single social work department should be created around either the children's departments or the health and welfare departments. Its strength, he argued, would lie in integrating a family welfare service with services for older people, those with mental ill health, the physically disabled. Others looked to unity as a family service. The report *Crime: A Challenge to Us All*, authored by Lord Longford (1905–2001), who was soon to be a minister in the Labour government that came to power in 1964, outlined a welfare-based juvenile justice system working closely with a local authority family service, an orientation generally supported by the Home Office. The preventive measures in the Children and Young Persons Act 1963 (see Chapter 10) also pointed to a family-based service with broader responsibilities, in essence unifying social work within an enlarged children's department.

At first, momentum lay with the notion of a family department but the discussion gradually widened, drawing in the interests of those working with the disabled and older people who had been overlooked in the debate. An ad hoc group formed, closely aligned with the Ministry of Health rather than the Home Office, and committed to a single social services department. Its most influential member was Richard Titmuss, an accomplished academic in social policy. He urged in a lecture in 1965 that a family service, no matter how widely defined, would not be able to respond to all clients; he specifically mentioned those with mental health problems, migrants, isolated older people, unmarried mothers and others who would hesitate before approaching a 'family department'. Nor, he argued, would a family department have room for residential and domiciliary services which all clients would draw on (Titmuss 1968). He proposed that social services departments should be created around the services to be provided and not around 'categories of clients or particular fragments of need' (as quoted in Cooper 1983: 63).

This idea for a generic service department was picked up by the National Institute for Social Work which had been created in 1961 with funds from the Ministry of Health and the Joseph Rowntree Memorial Trust as a kind of national staff college for training social workers and administrators. It provided the base for the ad hoc group lobbying for a single department (Cooper op cit.). That the ensuing debate was vehement gives us a sense of how much was perceived to be at stake at the time. Three matters were interlinked: (i) the most effective way to rearrange social services, with rising costs an important consideration; (ii) improving the quality of the services for those who used them; (iii) meeting the professional aspirations of social workers.

The idea of generic social work was further buttressed by the Younghusband Report (1959) which called for the introduction of all purpose social workers into local authorities. A new general training course would provide a qualification for the untrained welfare and mental welfare officers who would make up the majority of such workers and bring them up to the level of child care officers or psychiatric social workers. (Her inquiry had found that 89 per cent of social workers in the local authority sector were unqualified.) The general social worker, the report argued, would undertake a range of tasks in mental health, arranging the care and after-care of the sick, casework with families and in arranging care for older people (ibid: 10–12).

The Seebohm Committee and its report

To help settle the conflict, government appointed a committee of enquiry to be chaired by Frederic (later Lord) Seebohm with a brief to review the organization and responsibilities of local authority personal social services in England and Wales, and to 'consider what changes are desirable to secure an effective family service'. Membership of the committee became contentious as the then Ministry of Health and the Home Office jockeyed for influence, and from the start there were concerns that the National Institute for Social Work (NISW), which favoured the notion of a single generic department, was over-represented. Seebohm himself was chair of NISW, while other committee members were drawn from NISW staff.

The committee took a range of testimony – from social work organizations, local government officials, children's officers and academics but, unthinkable today, did not seek out users' views. Turf wars between the Home Office, which had oversight of the children's departments and thus was pushing for a family service, and the Ministry of Health (soon to be merged with Social Security) which had oversight of services for those with disability, mental health problems and older people, deepened the conflict. Inevitably this rivalry became mixed up with the substantive issues themselves. With the Seebohm Committee due to report shortly, the pot was stirred in part through the proposal in mid-1968 to launch community development projects in areas of inner-city decline under the auspices of the Home Office. While some scepticism was expressed about the unprecedented combative nature of the proposed projects at the Home Office itself, not least by the Home Secretary Jim Callaghan, ministers did see them as a useful tool to ensure that the Home Office would be the centre of urban social services and the children's departments as principal provider. Thus did the long-standing rivalry between Callaghan and Richard Crossman, Minister of Health, come to focus on which of them would have control over the new social services departments (Philpot 1977).

The principal social work organizations reached agreement on the shape of a single social services department. In this they received informal help from the Seebohm Committee itself which asked for evidence under clearly prescribed headings, and the social work organizations in their evidence brought the concept of a unitary organization well to the fore (Hall 1976: 47, 60).

The Standing Conference of Organizations of Social Workers offered its own evidence but could not disguise the fact that serious disagreement existed among its members on some of the issues, in particular on whether probation should be included within the new department (in the end it was not). Differences of approach also surfaced. The Association of Psychiatric Social Workers, always alert to protecting its elite status, welcomed

> a more flexible approach to treatment of social problems [but did] not subscribe to the concept of an all-purpose social worker...specialisation is essential to the advance of knowledge.... Furthermore, it is neither possible nor desirable for one person to be familiar with all aspects of legislation and administrative detail in relation to the many problems which affect clients....
>
> (quoted in Hall 1976: 51)

Report of the Committee on Local Authority and Allied Personal Social Services, 1968 (Seebohm Report)

The Seebohm Committee made the following recommendations:

- A comprehensive approach to the problems of individuals, families and their communities through the establishment in each local authority of a social services committee and a director of social services.
- Prevention, partnership, the role of the voluntary sector and the importance of harnessing the strengths of communities themselves were all emphasized.
- Continuity of care: the committee was against dividing social services by client group because it disrupted continuity of care to families and fragmented the profession.
- Generic training for all social workers.
- The new service would be family centred rather than 'symptom centred', and a family's needs should be 'served as far as possible by a single social worker'.

Social worker organizations lobbied hard for implementation of the recommendations by government. The Seebohm Implementation Action Group (SIAG), chaired by Tom White, then deputy children's officer for Lancashire and head of the Association of Child Care Officers, and Keith Bilton as secretary, worked tirelessly for the report to be legislated in full, at a time when, in 1969, the Labour government's enthusiasm for reform seemed to waver. Speaker's Notes laid out the case for activists to use as they fanned out across the country. The Notes rebutted the arguments against the 'monolithic' department and addressed the issue of genericism head on. While acknowledging that, in the past, significant progress had been made through specialist organizations 'at this point in time most progress will come from greater integration. It did not mean that everyone in a social service department would immediately drop what they were doing and undertake entirely different work. With careful preparation the transition should be followed by the release of time and energy through a more rational approach to the work' (SIAG, n.d.: C1).

The Local Authority Social Services Act

The Local Authority Social Services Act 1970 gave local authorities the duty to provide social services in England and Wales. While not defining social work (the Seebohm Committee did not either), the Act specified social services functions: child care, care of older and disabled people and care of those with mental health problems. Children's departments were abolished and their functions merged with mental welfare, education welfare and children's homes inside the new, vastly enlarged departments. It is important to recognize that both the Act and the Seebohm Committee Report itself were primarily about the organization of services. The fundamental debates about what social work should achieve largely took place *after* the formation of the new departments.

Tom White gives an account of the early days in the new departments

Tom White had been active within the Association of Child Care Officers in the early stages of his career, and as president of ACCO had been vigorous in lobbying for the Seebohm Implementation Action Group. On 1 August 1970 he was appointed director of the new social services department in Coventry, the first director to be appointed in the country, some eight months before authorities were legally obliged to do so. In his memoirs he writes of the promise and challenges of his early days in charge.

Coventry took the opportunity to maximize the advantage of bringing together all the 'social services' of the authority, going much further than the new Act made a statutory necessity. As a consequence the new Social Services Department incorporated the previously small separate Children's and Welfare Departments, the mental health services (including 'mental handicap' services from the Health Department), Sheltered Housing, including the wardens from the Housing Department and Education Welfare Officers from the Education Department. Together they created a large

> department – soon to grow into the second largest in the City in terms of staff (over 2000) and budget.
>
> Among the staff far too many 'poor law' attitudes persisted and often great ingenuity was put into finding ways of saying 'no' because of departmental convenience or cost rather than a genuine attempt to meet the needs of the client. In many parts of the service little ambition or imagination was shown, yet I soon discovered that there were many extremely able individuals who only needed to be enthused and encouraged to ensure real improvement in our services.
>
> (White 2011: 54–5)

Under the Social Work (Scotland) Act 1968, Scottish reorganization was more comprehensive than that in England. It gave local authorities a general duty to promote social welfare; it integrated the probation service into the local authority social work service; and it introduced at the same time a more radical reform of juvenile justice than had been introduced in England and Wales by the separate and never-to-be-fully-implemented Children and Young Persons Act 1969 (see Chapter 11). It was also achieved more quickly.

The generic department takes shape

The creation of the large department should be placed in context. It was a time of general belief in large-scale programmes that would deliver greater equality and fairness. Large council house estates – Park Hill in Sheffield in the early 1960s and Thamesmead in London in the late 1960s – offer a parallel example. While the Local Authority Social Services Act 1970 was passed during the last months of power of the Labour government, it was implemented after the election in June 1970 by the Conservative government. Keith Joseph, minister for social services, oversaw significant expansion in the early 1970s promising a funding increase of some 10 per cent *per year*. Only after the Conservative defeats of 1974 (there were two elections that year) did he come to review his work in government and become more closely wedded to the anti-bureaucratic, free market philosophy for which he is now known.

The new departments integrated very different social work activities – with different legal frameworks, organizational concerns and skills. People who could assist in the transition could be found at different levels in the hierarchy and by no means automatically at senior levels. The fact was that all levels of staff had to deal with problems which went beyond their basic experiences, involving a mix of policy and operational issues. In addition, financial and legal expertise had to be drawn in as well as strategic planning expertise. Among the directors of the new departments, Tom White was the first but eventually not alone in seeing the need to develop departmental research capacity and to invest in training (White 2011).

The new departments had to deliver services across wide areas such as the shire counties and large populations in urban centres. They had to devise ways to integrate the comparatively small children's departments with the larger welfare departments. The former operated with flat hierarchies – a team of child care workers and child home managers responsible to the children's office whereas the latter, which had to deliver comparatively routine services, were hierarchical. While a flat organizational hierarchy had been effective for social casework, it was not so for large departments; centralized control required a layer of middle management to facilitate the linking of these concerns (Hill 2000: 160).

The premise of the social services department was that it created a 'single door' through which people and families with various needs could go for assistance. This resulted in unprecedented levels of demand for social work services that required rationing to take place at lower levels of the organization. The conflicting ideals between universalism and genericism on the one hand and selectivity and specialization on the other left many unresolved tensions for front-line staff to manage (Ellis et al. 1999). In the face of the broad social hopes embodied in the Seebohm vision and widely shared by managers and practitioners, considerable discretion had to be given to front-line staff and team leaders as first-tier managers. In a period when operational guidelines were sparse, if they existed at all, and the notion of performance measurement non-existent, ambiguous policy objectives could be met only by giving front-line staff considerable scope for decision making.

With this relative autonomy came a new kind of pressure. Satyamurti's analysis of a single social services department shortly after it was formed found that the average caseload for field social workers, 44, was no greater than those carried by child care officers in the former children's department and was substantially less than that of the medical social workers and welfare officers who also became part of the department. Although she established that the field social workers were wrong in believing that the stress levels of their job came from the number of cases they were responsible for, she identified other pressures: location in area offices, with clients walking into the office on a more regular basis, reduced administrative support, staff shortages and increased statutory duties arising from the Children and Young Persons Act 1969 (see Chapter 10) and the Chronically Sick and Disabled Act 1970 (see Chapter 11) (Satyamurti 1981: 47–8).

The social work team offered some buttress against such pressures, the source of solidarity, support, and mentoring. Strong in its cohesion there was pronounced resistance to any differentiation within the group. Team members were aware of the great responsibilities shouldered by each of them – child protection, compulsory admission to mental hospital, where to place the disabled child when very old parents could no longer cope. Satyamurti observed:

> The emphasis on the lack of differentiation within the team carried the implicit message that all team members were the same, and there-fore when mistakes were made, or tragedies occurred it could be felt by the social worker concerned that this was something that 'could happen to anyone'. This emphasis on everyone being in the same situation was a collective means of offsetting the isolation and the anxiety that derived from the privatised [that is, individual] nature of the work.
>
> (ibid.: 63).

Creation of the British Association of Social Workers

The common experience of lobbying for implementation of the Seebohm Re-port brought the various social work professional associations together in what proved to be an effective working relationship within the Standing Conference of Organizations of Social Workers. Many of these associations had their own lengthy and proud history but saw the need now, in the wake of the creation of the single social services department, to give organizational voice to a com-mon vision of social work. Sporadic attempts in the past to do so had been only partially successful, such as the British Federation of Social Workers formed in 1936 which changed its name to the Association of Social Work (ASW) in 1951. With its widely read journal *Case Conference*, the ASW pressed for the foundation of a single professional association. This was duly formed in April 1970, combining eight organizations: the Association of Child Care Officers, the Association of Family Caseworkers, the Association of Psychiatric Social Workers, the Association of Moral Welfare Workers, the Institute of Medical Social Workers, the Society of Mental Welfare Officers, and the Association of Social Workers itself (see Figure 7.2). The National Association of Probation Officers chose not to join although it had participated in the discussions and viewed itself as a social work organization.

The major issue that BASW confronted from the outset was whether to have open membership. The psychiatric social workers and almoners worked closely with the medical settings in which they were largely based, while child care officers and probation officers, for whom qualification was not a requirement, worked in local government settings. The first group, based in large urban areas, strongly defended a membership based on qualification whereas the second advocated open membership for unqualified staff and

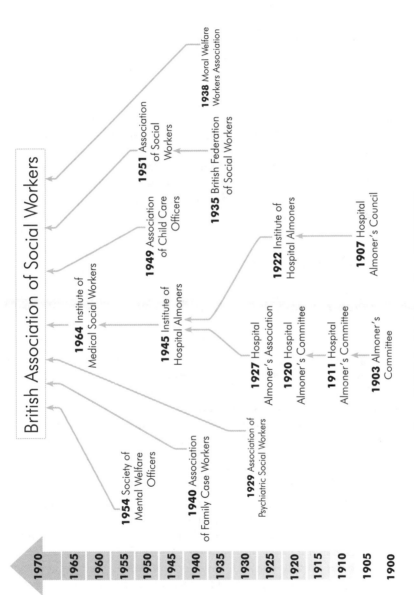

Figure 7.2 Unity at last: Formation of BASW 1970

British Association of Social Workers

1970
1965
1960
1955
1950
1945
1940
1935
1930
1925
1920
1915
1910
1905
1900

1954 Society of Mental Welfare Officers

1940 Association of Family Case Workers

1929 Association of Psychiatric Social Workers

1964 Institute of Medical Social Workers

1945 Institute of Hospital Almoners

1927 Hospital Almoner's Association

1920 Hospital Almoner's Committee

1911 Hospital Almoner's Committee

1903 Almoner's Committee

1951 Association of Social Workers

1935 British Federation of Social Workers

1949 Association of Child Care Officers

1922 Institute of Hospital Almoners

1907 Hospital Almoner's Council

1938 Moral Welfare Workers Association

emergent radical social workers (see next chapter), making the charge that BASW was elitist. These divisions ran deep. As Payne (2002: 972) put it, 'Every annual general meeting was rent by the debate about this issue, until "open membership" was approved in 1978'. Even so, it was not until 1987 that those who had obtained the Certificate in Social Service (CSS) – a qualification for social work assistants, home care organizers and managers of residential units – were admitted to full membership.

Soon after its foundation BASW launched a monthly magazine, *Social Work Today*, to replace the various journals of the older professional associations such as *Medical Social Work, Mental Welfare News* or the *Bulletin of the Association of Moral Welfare Workers*. It became a weekly in 1974 to keep up with a new rival *Community Care* (see Chapter 8). There were persistent questions however over BASW's control of editorial policy and the degree to which it could make criticisms of its parent organization (Philpot 1991). (Despite BASW relinquishing full control in 1988 the magazine was eventually bought out by Reed Business Publishing in the 1990s and closed.)

Unifying social work method

As conceptualizations of casework became more varied, and the psychodynamic model began to fragment and lose its dominance in the early 1970s, the discussion of methods in social work went in two different directions at the same time.

The first sought to find unity of method, to provide, as a leading textbook of the time put it, 'a common set of principles and concepts which *all* social workers could use in dealing with social problems as they are manifest in a single individual, group or a community' (Specht and Vickery 1977: 15). The aim of those promoting a unitary or integrated method was to equip the social worker, now practising in an open-ended field and having to deal with a range of social and personal problems, with an adaptable perspective 'that allowed them to plan, implement and evaluate their practice in the context of that totality' (ibid.: 25). Fundamentally integrating methods would help social workers make choices and communicate more effectively. Today we might cast it in terms of generic, adaptable skills such as learning how to combine functions, to draw on evidence, to create networked communities of practice, and generate inclusive visioning.

In actuality the unitary method, based on a modified systems approach developed in the United States, allowed for specialization in practice – such as social casework, group work or community work – but also recognized what it called 'the generalist professional' who would have a mixture of roles – as enabler and coordinator of teams of para-professionals, the mediator between client groups and service organizations, and the resource developer (Specht and Vickery 1977: 239). In this it was remarkably forward looking.

The second was to formalize the variety of approaches that emerged from casework as a suite of methods: crisis intervention, behavioural and cognitive behavioural work, and task-centred work. They became the subject of many a textbook variously defining the 'approaches', 'methods' or 'theories' of social work over a thirty-year period. Most were developed outside social work: crisis intervention was developed by two psychiatrists, Erich Lindemann and Gerald Caplan, in the 1960s, and cognitive behavioural therapy by another psychiatrist Aaron Beck also in the 1960s. Both approaches had wide application and were used by all manner of therapists in addition to social workers.

A plurality of methods led to several difficulties. It was difficult to prove whether they 'worked', and social workers in any case were notoriously slow in evaluating their methods or even submitting them to external evaluation. Claiming to have different methods also allowed social workers to choose the one that most interested them, with no evidence to hand as to whether it was effective. The multitude of methods were also difficult for clients to understand, particularly by those users who had largely practical problems on their mind and did not view the social worker as a therapeutic agent. Of the major methods, only task-centred work could be said to have originated within social work, emerging from Reid and Epstein's work (1972). While durable – appearing in university syllabuses for decades – these methods were progressively hedged by notions of the 'reflective practitioner' and 'practice theories' which gave greater prominence to the personal models based on workers' accumulating experiences (Hardiker and Barker 1981; Schön 1983).

Summary

- Experiences in the Second World War shaped the formation of the welfare state and social work's position within it.
- Social casework became the dominant method of social work but produced critics as well.
- In 1968 the Seebohm Committee, after much deliberation, recommended setting up a single social services department in each local authority, combining all services in one.
- BASW was formed as a single professional organization to represent social workers.
- By the 1960s a range of 'methods' emerged as social casework began to lose its dominance.

Suggested reading

Cooper, J. (1983). *Creation of the British Personal Social Services 1962–1974*. London: Heinemann.

Hall, P. (1976). *Reforming the Welfare: The Politics of Change in the Personal Social Services*. London: Heinemann.

Younghusband, E. (1978). *Social Work in Britain, 1950–1975*. London: George Allen & Unwin.

8 Radical Voices, Turbulent Times

In the 1970s, social work faced severe tests from inside and outside the profession. Its conduct and purpose came under close public scrutiny – and for the first time it faced criticism and outright hostility. This chapter examines:

- the radical voices that emerged from within social work;
- the debate over whether social work was a profession or an occupation and part of the trade union movement;
- the attacks from the political right which questioned whether social workers were needed at all;
- the move to see clients as fellow citizens as principles of due process begin to apply to social work decision making.

'The party is over'

The economic and currency crisis that came to a head in 1976, requiring a bailout by the International Monetary Fund, marked a profound change of context for the public sector in general and social work in particular. Compared with the cuts in local government in 2011, the expenditure standstill envisaged by the Labour government of 1976 seems modest. But relative to expectations at the time, with regular annual growth of social services budgets of some 10 per cent in the early 1970s, it was a shock. It is difficult for us now to imagine that there was once a time when social service budgets were adjusted (upwards) to meet declared need as the financial year progressed. The imposition of 'cash limits', that is, having to work within a fixed annual budget, seemed an affront to social justice. When Anthony Crosland, Labour minister of local government, said 'the party is over' in 1975, he was greeted with a mixture of outrage and disbelief within the public sector and crystallized within social work a trend that had been developing for some time: radicalism.

Anthony Crosland announces imminent expenditure cuts in local government
In a speech in Manchester on a May 1975, the minister for local government, Anthony Crosland, said: For the next few years times will not be normal. Perhaps people have used the words 'economic crisis' too often in the past. They have shouted 'wolf, wolf' when the animal was more akin to a rather disagreeable Yorkshire terrier. But not now. The crisis that faces us is infinitely more serious than any of the crises we have faced over the past 20 years. . . . With its usual spirit of patriotism and its tradition of service to the community's needs, it [local government] is coming to realize that, for the time being at least, the party is over. . . . We are not calling for a headlong retreat. But we are calling for a standstill. *Source: The Times*, 10 May 1975.

Emergence of radical social work

The period of radical social work's influence was fairly short. The movement could be said to have begun with the publication of the journal *Case Con* in 1972, hit a peak of influence in the mid-1970s, but to have lost that influence by the early 1980s. How widely shared the radical vision was among practitioners is difficult to say – it was significant although never a majority viewpoint.

Radical social work, often drawing on a Marxist perspective, argued for solidarity with clients on the basis that both they and social workers were oppressed – practitioners by the large bureaucratic organizations within which they worked and clients by the class structure and poverty to which their lives were condemned. Radical social workers sought to:

- extend the range of benefits for claimants as part of an anti-poverty strategy;
- move beyond casework to expand clients' political awareness and tackle structural sources of inequality and social injustice, including community action;
- link with claimants' unions and welfare rights organizations.

Radicals regarded their own departments as oppressive because of their size and bureaucracy, with senior managers unncessarily focused on cost efficiencies.

Why did radical social work emerge in the early 1970s?

Radical social work can be viewed as part of a general move to the left within some white-collar professions as they became aware of the gulf between them and the people they ostensibly served. There were parallel developments among city planners, lawyers and architects. Radicals in general understood that society rested on exploitation of the working class by those who controlled the means of production and that antagonism between social classes was the prime characteristic of society that, depending on the outcome of that struggle, produced social change. Militancy was in the air, and the extent of social conflict was evident in the miners' strikes of 1973–74, the last of which led indirectly to the fall of the Conservative government, and in the broadly supported strike of women dressmakers – most of whom were south Asian – at the Grunwick plant in London in 1976.

Were social workers working class or from the professional middle class? This was a complicated question. Corrigan and Leonard, in one of the more perceptive and influential texts of the time, put it this way:

> although they [social workers] are in fact merely selling their own labour, their function as part of the ideological State apparatus ... gives them a clear role on behalf of the bourgeoisie. However, an understanding of this and realization that one cannot be a neutral professional between the opposing classes may have the effect of enabling radical social workers to begin to perform some political role, albeit a small one, within the working class and labour movement.
>
> (Corrigan and Leonard 1978: 84)

They were cautioning social workers against seeing themselves as fully fledged members of the working class and to be realistic about their class location. On the other hand, they argued that social workers were exposed to anti-capitalist influence and were at the heart of a major contradiction of the welfare state: as agents of social policy they were attempting the impossible, namely trying to soften the increasingly severe dislocations of capitalism. Awareness of their position could enable social workers to undertake an oppositionist political role, one in which they have more autonomy than the formal coercive institutions of the state such as the police and army. Social workers, Corrigan and Leonard argued, may be engaged in struggle like their clients, but did so on a '*subordinate* basis, that is, it was not experienced as gaining power, it was not experienced as *choice* to do something or another; nearly all struggle is experienced as "not letting *them* get away with it"' (ibid.: 88).

Case Con manifesto 1972

'CASE CON is an organisation of social workers (in the broadest sense), attempting to give an answer to the contradictions that we face. Case Con offers no magic solutions, no way in which you can go to work tomorrow and practice some miraculous new form of social work which does meet the needs of your "clients". It would be nice if there were such an easy answer, but we believe that the problems and frustrations we face daily are inextricably linked to the society we live in, and that we can only understand what needs to be done if we understand how the welfare state, of which social services are a part, has developed, and what pressures it is subject to. It is the purpose of this manifesto to trace briefly this development, to see how it affects us and our relationships to the rest of society, and above all to start working out what we can do about it.

'The welfare state was set up partly in response to working-class agitation and mainly to stabilize the upheavals generated by wartime conditions. It was recognised that improvements in the living conditions of workers helped provide capitalism with a more efficient work force and could nip militancy in the bud. Furthermore, the threat of withdrawal of benefits under certain conditions (being on strike or cohabiting, for example) could be a useful technique of social control. . . .

. . .

'It was also decided [by government] to utilize the resources of the community itself to tackle social problems at both an individual and a community level. Thus, a new category of worker was proposed to discover and promote these resources within the community and to emphasise the importance of people doing things for themselves rather than depending on the corporation or on the government. This can be seen also in recent changes in legislation dealing with criminal offenders, for example, community service orders and intermediate treatment schemes. The encouragement of voluntary organizations was another important facet of the new strategy, and official dependence on such organizations as Child Poverty Action Group and Shelter is increasing. Even claimants' unions and squatters have been successfully co-opted by the state.'

Source: http://www.radical.org.uk/barefoot/casecon.htm (accessed 9 October 2010).

Discussion point   Does the Case Con manifesto have any relevance today?

The Case Con manifesto was written in 1972 for the launch of the radical social work magazine (in which the youthful Steve Bell, now long established as the political cartoonist for the *Guardian* newspaper, published his first cartoons). What parts of it do you think still have relevance today? What parts do not?

Social work as profession or trade union?

Radical social work in its anti-professional stance triggered a wider debate: did social work's future lie as a fully fledged profession or as an occupation organized within a trade union? While social workers had been trying to achieve professional status for virtually the entire twentieth century – a goal, as we have seen, that had largely eluded them – by the 1970s the view that social work was an occupation whose conditions of work would be most effectively defended by trade union membership extended beyond those who were radical leaning. In general, professional status was thought to be elitist, distancing practitioners from those they served and with whom they wanted to be in alliance. Other critics of professionalism noted the inadvertently harmful effects of professional service, prone to error and negligence but with the capacity to cover these up. Ivan Illich, whose writings were popular at the time, called this 'social iatrogenesis' – the inadvertent harm that ensued as people were moved from one environment to another (Illich 1975).

Trade union membership offered an alternative affiliation to professional association that would both obtain better pay and conditions and offer practitioners organizational agency in changing society. As trade unionists there were no difficulties over who should not be included: the more the better. Qualified social workers alongside unqualified social workers, social work assistants, home helps (home care assistants), cleaners and other domestic staff provided a forceful alliance for better services and fairer deals for clients. But with trade unionism came calls – at times militant calls – for improved working conditions and salaries. Specific demands as put forward by the National Association for Local Government Officers (NALGO) were for regrading fieldworkers' pay, enhanced payments for 'standby' or being on-call out of hours, and for local negotiations between employers and unions.

It is important to bear in mind that the influence of trade unions generally was far greater in the 1970s than it is now; overall union membership was at an historic high and unions – from the miners, to car workers, print workers, and many others – regularly displayed their willingness to take industrial action in pursuit of pay claims. In general, shop floor leaders such as shop stewards were much more powerful than now, with local, unofficial or 'wildcat' strikes far more common. Social work and residential care staff were not immune to this outlook.

Two major trade unions represented social workers in the 1970s. The majority were in NALGO, but in certain areas the National Union of Public Employees (NUPE) also represented social workers – and was the more militant by comparison. The left of these unions viewed local authorities less as organs of popular local will and more as administrators of national government policy; councillors, the thinking ran, although elected, were not responsible to the electorate in the same way as union negotiators or officials were to their members.

There was therefore a fundamental conflict between those social workers who sought to become part of a fully fledged profession with a powerful and influential professional body regulating and representing its members, and those who thought trade unionism was the most effective, inclusive way forward.

The National Union of Public Employees in Birmingham

The largest NUPE branch for social workers was in Birmingham; it combined social workers, qualified and unqualified (see next box), home helps and a range of domiciliary and care assistant staff. By the end of 1977 the branch had trebled its membership over four years to a total of 2,150, making it the largest trade union within the social services department in the city. Shop stewards were accorded an influential role: they consulted the workforce, demanded (and obtained) time off with pay for branch committee members, and the right to hold union meetings in work time.

In Birmingham the fieldworkers and residential workers who dominated the social services branch were anti-hierarchical, suspicious of co-option by senior management, and in favour of rank and file power. In their campaigns they sought:

- a single pay grade increase across the board for all social service employees;
- a pay increase of over 10 percent – which was then the annual rate of inflation;
- for those on training courses, to be seconded without loss of salary;
- 30 days' minimum annual leave, nearly twice the current 18 days;
- time off in lieu (TOIL) on an hour-for-hour basis specifically mentioning that weekends spent away with social services children should equate to 35–40 hours TOIL.

From the branch perspective, social workers functioned within a fractious, discontented environment, with individual homes and individual area offices in dispute at various times. NUPE saw that considerable potential power lay with the residential workers, community care workers, cooks and drivers who distributed essential supplies to care homes. Thus, working with these 'lower status' occupations furthered not only working-class solidarity but also a link with powerful allies. In the late 1970s, during the last years of the Labour government but with the Conservative Party in power in Birmingham, the union fought any kind of pay restraint or pay policy as well as the city-wide freeze on recruitment and the closure of residential homes.

The branch newsletter for January 1978 gives an indication of its objectives. Under the headline 'Staff Take Control', the article is indicative of the issues then being seriously debated:

How far should workers control the decision made about their work? Should workers pick their own bosses? How much of workers' lives should management manage? How much does higher management know about the daily situations that workers face?

These question and others have recently been aired ... where NUPE-led workforces conducted interviews of the candidates for the post of Area Manager. In the process, some common assumptions were put to the test. The further up the management ladder you go, the bigger the decisions which are made, but the bigger, too becomes the distance from the client. We always assume that management has a right to make these decisions and that part of our job is just to carry them out. But is it really right and proper that important individual decisions should be made without ever seeing the client, or Departmental policy formed by people who never come in contact with the public in their daily work? ... No-one ever suggests that someone should be responsible to the community of clients for the fact that resources are insufficient ... because in this kind of hierarchical set-up, the clients come at the bottom of the ladder, and have no power to ask questions or make decisions.

('Staff Take Control', *NUPE Journal (Birmingham Social Services Branch)* No. 7, January 1978, p. 3)

Demands on unqualified social workers in the West Midlands

The number of qualified social workers within the department in the 1970s could be quite small, and unqualified social workers were expected to take on heavy responsibilities from the beginning. When Martin Thomas joined a West Midlands team as an unqualified social worker in 1974 the other eight team members were also unqualified – only the team manager held a qualification. New social workers were unprotected. As he recounted: '... the practice was to offload a few cases [from each social worker] to any new recruit. Within the first couple of weeks I was given around 25 cases of a mixture of child care, mental health and adult cases – many extremely complex and stressful and often cases that the previous worker had found difficult I suspect. Within six weeks I was made an "approved social worker" because as the area manager put it, I seemed to be "reasonably sensible" ' (Martin Thomas, pers. comm.).

In the view of its largely youthful membership, the welfare state was a system in which social work and the social services department played a prominent part in cooling dissent and mollifying the population of have-nots. Thus radical social work argued that both social workers and their clients were enmeshed in a system of state welfare. But radical social work also acknowledged that there were contradictions in wielding authority within and on behalf of the state sector, on the one hand, and promoting radical social change on the other. The dilemma for radical practitioners was clear: how can social work responsibilities be carried out with integrity on behalf of a state system when

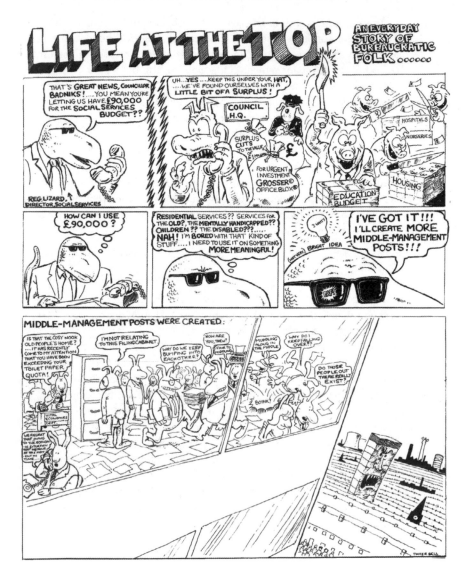

Steve Bell Cartoons: Steve Bell, well-known political cartoonist for the Guardian, drew several cartoons for the NUPE branch newsletter in the late 1970s under the pen-name 'Tinkerbell'. They perfectly capture the view that senior social services management and Birmingham Council leaders worked closely together to bureaucratise the service and control practitioners on the ground.

The first cartoon appeared in the Birmingham Branch NUPE Newsletter of March 1978, the second in the Newsletter of May 1978.

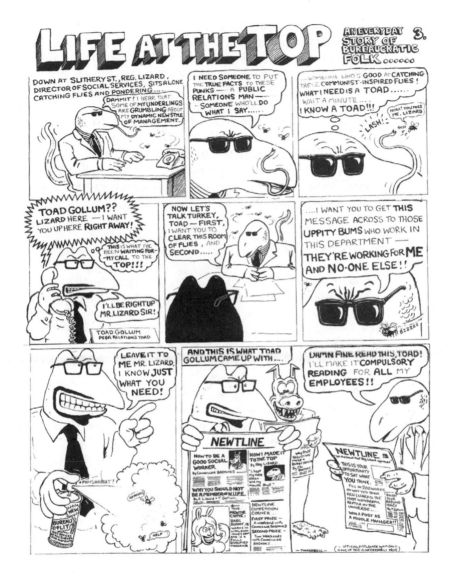

that very system is deemed to prop up exploitation? The dilemma was never fully surmounted as radical practitioners themselves perhaps would admit; often the response could be no more than the admonition 'to work against the system from within the system'.

Social workers are so placed, however, that they have the capacity to observe and understand the nature of these contradictions. As one of the most thoughtful Marxist social work educators put it: 'Social workers, although situated in a largely oppressive organizational and professional context, have the potential for recognizing these contradictions and, through working at the point of interaction between people and their social environment, of helping to increase the control by people over economic and political structures' (Leonard 1975: 55). Social work in capitalist society, he argued, aims to diminish individual suffering caused substantially by the consequences of economic production. The key task is education – to develop a critical consciousness in clients of their oppression and to link with others on this basis. In this, radical social work moved closer to the approach of Paulo Freire, the radical Brazilian educator, based on 'conscientization' through dialogue and helping users to obtain even small gains in control over the systems within which they are caught; gains upon which they can base further learning.

The social workers' strike

The only major strike – ever – by social workers took place in 1978–79. The union, NALGO, did not call out social workers nationally but left it to individual branches to decide. In the event, only a handful of local authorities – 15 out of 143 – went on strike, among them Newcastle, Cheshire, Liverpool, Birmingham and Leeds, and several London boroughs such as Tower Hamlets, Hackney, Greenwich, Lewisham and Southwark. Craig Cawthorn (2010) has noted the irony that strikes took place in some of the most progressive authorities with directors at the helm who were largely sympathetic to the strikers' objectives, such as Maurice Speed in Cheshire and Brian Roycroft in Newcastle. Elsewhere, senior management was less sympathetic, as in Liverpool and Birmingham.

The broad case made by the unions reflected the kinds of things that Satyamurti (see previous chapter) and others had observed regarding working conditions within the social services departments. It pointed to the upheaval in service since the late 1960s, not only in reorganization but also in additional legal duties that social workers were now responsible for that had come with the Children and Young Persons Act 1969, Chronically Sick and Disabled Act 1970, and the Children Act 1975. NALGO also argued that there was insufficient pay for being 'on call' through nights and weekends, when it was customary for social workers to drive out on their own to deal with a nighttime crisis – an adolescent at the local police station whose parents refused to have him home, assessing a child at risk or compulsorily admitting a person under the Mental Health Act 1959. (The reader today should remember that in the 1970s these were tasks that all social workers, including the newest, would undertake.)

The NALGO branches that went on strike – and the NUPE branches in several of the striking authorities – were pressing for:

- substantial pay increases based on a regrading of their work;
- a pay structure that reflected career advancement;
- enhanced bands of pay for overtime;
- local pay negotiations.

The local authorities as employers found the last objective the most difficult to concede and argued instead for a national framework within which local negotiations could take place to adjust pay to local conditions. On several occasions the employers would assert that they were negotiating in good faith and wanted strikers to call off their action as a result; the strikers just as regularly rejected such calls until negotiations had been concluded. Significantly, social workers received full pay from NALGO throughout the strike and so did not endure any hardship. That was not the case for NUPE members who relied on donations from their union and from NALGO branches.

The dispute came to a phased end as successive local authorities settled without signed deals with their social workers. The final agreement, probably available earlier, included:[1]

- No local deal on pay though some flexibility in local negotiations on particular issues was obtained.
- Significant pay increases introduced by some local authorities through the introduction of a three-tier career pay grade with unqualified staff on level 1, qualified social workers on level 2 and social workers with substantial experience of handling complex cases on level 3. Many authorities reserved level 3 for senior social workers with supervisory responsibilities and placed a limit on their number. Other authorities such as Cheshire County Council did not limit the number of level 3 social workers or demand supervisory tasks but did introduce a procedure by which those on level 2 could only progress to level 3 by demonstrating through interview and portfolio of competence that they could manage a complex caseload. Nevertheless, post-strike there was the presumption that many social workers would move swiftly if not immediately to the level 3 attracting the higher pay.
- An additional two pay increments based on 'local conditions' were available to social workers at all levels who worked in areas of high deprivation. Some authorities, such as Cheshire, applied this selectively, but others – Liverpool, Tower Hamlets and Newcastle – applied it across the board.
- While the establishment of out-of-hours emergency duty teams had been raised by strikers in various authorities, such teams only emerged later as the result of separate national negotiations.
- Newly qualified staff were to receive a protected caseload.

Although only a fraction of social workers had gone on strike the new pay and conditions spread quickly across the local authority sector and was not confined to those authorities that had been on strike.

What the long-term effects of the strike were is an interesting question to consider. Whether it ushered in change or was itself a symptom of change already under way is uncertain. Some on the right wing of the Conservative Party saw the strike as proof positive that social workers were not needed at all. Nobody died as a consequence they argued, or experienced increased distress (Brewer and Lait 1980). Twenty-five years later there was still substantial disagreement among former strikers themselves over what had been achieved. Some questioned whether it had been right to strike at all, leaving vulnerable clients on their own, while others thought the strike had damaged the reputation of social work (Community Care 2003).

Yet others pointed to the improvement in wages and conditions and to the fact that NALGO began to see social workers as an important, articulate part of its membership. Wider issues about the direction of social work did receive an airing as social workers began to look hard at how to extend a progressive vision of social work, one that explicitly worked for social justice but within the parameters of stipulated responsibilities, in for example community social work. (See below.)

The trade union movement on the whole, however, was on the eve of dramatic loss of membership and influence following the election of the Conservative government in 1979. In perhaps no more than two years, even radicals came to see that the capacity of social work, as part of the trade union movement, to effect social change was diminished. When the miners went on strike in 1983, social work departments in the mining districts of England, Wales and Scotland worked hard to offset the hardship that miners and their families were experiencing, but they did so as professionals, using tools at their disposal. By then, secondary picketing had been outlawed in the Employment Act 1980, in the second year of the Thatcher government, but in any case there was little appetite within NALGO to engage in any sympathetic action. This compelled radicals to realign their thinking in directions more congruent with the day-to-day tasks, roles and means that social work actually had at its disposal. Not a few radicals and strike leaders migrated into management posts, some to emerge in the 1990s as consultants or New Labour theorists.

Inside BASW, the strike caused upheaval. BASW did not endorse the right to strike until August 1978, yet two years earlier its conference had voted to set up its own trade union for social workers. As BASW general secretary Chris Andrews said: 'So long as the identity of a social worker is fused with that of a local government officer it is unlikely that social work will be able to develop as an independent discipline' (quoted in Weinstein 1984). With a membership of 10,000, BASW saw itself as a credible alternative to NALGO, which it regarded as a bureaucratic, even monopolistic, structure. BASW established the British

Union of Social Workers which was certified as a trade union in 1977. Few qualified social workers joined it, however, and following financial difficulties in the early 1980s the union combined with the small National Union of Social Workers to become the British Union of Social Work Employee (BUSWE). (In 2008 BUSWE formally joined Community – a small care-sector trade union – and continues to operate as a section within it.)

Community Care

In the absence of a recognized institution to which social workers could look to for support and authority one common platform for debate, the weekly magazine *Community Care*, played a vital role in forging common viewpoint and common agendas. Begun in 1974 it flowered throughout the last quarter of the twentieth century under the editorship of Terry Philpot with a readership in tens of thousands across field, residential and domiciliary social services. It widely promoted discussion of social work issues drawing on the expertise of practitioners, academics and journalists. Its activity went beyond the magazine itself, to include regular conferences, annual award ceremonies for innovative practice, a prestigious annual lecture, research monographs in association with Sheffield University, books on practice with noted publishers. It is difficult now, given the myriad of platforms for news and comment – blogs, on-line, tweets and social network sites – to understand how astonishing that level of activity was in giving voice to the plurality of viewpoints while acting as consistent advocate for social work itself.

Community Care leader October 11 1978

In the midst of the social work strike Terry Philpot, the new editor *Community Care* wrote one of his first leaders urging parity of pay for field and residential workers.

'If, as we have repeatedly stated, the case for paying field workers more is strong, then that is even more so for residential workers. It is nothing short of scandalous that (to offer recent examples from our own pages) a senior house-parent in a London observation and assessment centre is paid between £3,273 and £3,750 and sleep-in duty is required for only £2.30 a night. ...Unlike field workers, residential staffs cannot strike. To most of them such an idea is abhorrent. . . .

'A complete review must be established to offer a comprehensive view and solutions to pay in the social services. Not only would this give justice to both types of social worker and offer parity, it would also be a practical symbolic step in ensuring that residential work is part of the total continuum of care and not, as is often the case, just a poor, ill-nourished relation.'

Radical social work's legacy

In the 1970s the ideology of radical social work could be said to be an ortho-
dox leftism pushing for greater public expenditure and improved wages and
conditions for social workers while aguing that both social workers and their
clients were exploited by welfare state bureaucracies. As that vision foundered
on the rapidly diminishing power of the trade union movement in the early
1980s, other kinds of radical influences began to develop outside social work
but allied to it: the disability movement, mental health survivor movement,
feminist social work and anti-racist social work. All were to make their impact
in the coming decade, and the radicalism of the mid to late 1970s can be said
to have prepared the ground through its understanding of collective experiences embracing users and practitioners. This was an essential first step taken
by the radicalism of the 1970s and augmented with the forceful message from
user advocacy groups that social workers actually had a great deal of power
compared with users and that a critique of that power was a prerequisite for
progressive practice. Until that point, solidarity with clients was more talked
about than put into practice. A decade later, anti-racist and anti-discriminatory
social work would continue to gather strength – and in turn to be targeted by
the tabloid media as the epitome of 'political correctness'.

Community social work

Community social work adapted some of radical social work's interest in community development. Yet it had a different outlook and different aims, namely
to provide decentralized, neighbourhood-oriented systems of delivery focused
on a small geographical area. The approach was pioneered in, among other
places, Normanton, West Yorkshire, in the late1970s as 'patch' social work.

Patch work sidestepped the issue of solidarity with the trade union movement as the vehicle for social change. But it did pick up the radicals' enthusiasm for community work and kept geographical communities as a target for
intervention while at the same time trying to overcome the distance between
professional and client. It also developed concepts with which we are now familiar but which were then just coming into vogue: neighbourhood councils
as 'a forum for participation', councils setting up a 'participation committee',
calls for participatory structures and opening up the local authority's committee system to public involvement.

While radical social work often sought directly to change social and economic structures by raising the consciousness of users – bringing practitioners,
welfare claimants and trade unionists together as change agents – community
social work called on social workers to focus on strengthening informal social networks as key to providing care.[2] Community social work recognized
the capacity of networks and worked to bolster those networks or to bring
new networks to life where they were insufficient. Rather than focus on an

individual client and their immediate family it recognized that social problems arise in part through malfunctioning social networks (Hadley et al. 1987). In this community social work anticipated much of the later thinking on community participation and social capital.

The Barclay Report

In 1980 the Conservative government asked the National Institute of Social Work to undertake an independent enquiry to review the role and tasks of social workers in the local authority and voluntary sector in England and Wales. The report, known as the Barclay Report after the committee's chairperson Peter Barclay and published in 1982, aroused wide interest in England and Wales and in Scotland. It noted that many social workers were now embarrassed by the term 'social casework' and was clear that it was time for social work to move beyond the conventional three methods available to it: casework, group work and community work. In reviewing what social workers actually did across field teams, day centres and residential care, it found two main roles: *social care planning* – designing packages of care which required knowledge of local social networks – and *counselling* – to understand and plan with clients how to manage the practical and emotional realities facing them.

The report was notable for the case it made for community social work. Broadly, it argued that the great bulk of social care was provided within and by communities – family, friends, neighbours, local organizations. It defined community as 'a network, or networks, of informal relationships between people connected with each other by kinship, common interest, geographical proximity, friendship, occupation, or the giving and receiving of services – or various combinations of these'. Such networks, it argued, had the capacity to 'mobilise individual and collective responses to adversity' and called for social work to sustain networks and create them where they were absent (Barclay Committee 1982: 199).

The report met with a range of criticism that largely focused on the Committee's failure to confer professional status on social work. It did not recommend establishing a general council to regulate the profession and set standards – nor did it spell out sufficiently the specialness of social work in the eyes of these critics. Other criticisms focused on the lack of clarity around community social work – did it simply mean more *community-based* social services? Perhaps the main criticism, however, was that the Committee did not spell out what departmental structures would most effectively deliver these kinds of objectives (Thomas 1984).

With hindsight, many of these criticisms were misplaced and the report remains an important document in situating social work in our time. It was first to explain social care planning as part of the social work role. It also underscored the importance of working with ready partners and allied occupations across the day, domiciliary and residential care systems and foresaw the importance of voluntary organizations in delivering social care. It foreshadowed drawing on 'social capital' and the capacities stored in social relationships in a locality – whether 'networks for getting by' or 'getting ahead' – and called on social work to support and strengthen such networks. Its discussion of the importance of social work values inaugurated and widened what had previously been a topic of muted narrowness, while at the same time acknowledging that those values – compassion, understanding, sympathy, justice, equality and fairness – were not unique to social work. It explicitly rejected the notion that social work should be defined in terms of the values it espouses, rather than in terms of specific roles and tasks.

The Barclay Committee promotes community social work

'Our main reason for believing that such an approach [community social work] is now possible is that there has been a very general movement away from centralism and towards a belief in the capacity of ordinary people. This trend is seen already, or there is pressure for it to occur, in such diverse areas as party politics, discussion within trade unions, a disaffection with the older professions, the way some police forces are organized, in the management of rundown housing estates and in the move to decentralise authority in large industrial undertaking. People themselves are very generally less willing to tolerate the taking of decisions by remote authority which does not take account of circumstances affecting their neighourhoods or communities of interest.'

Source: Barclay Commitee 1982: 204.

Community social work – the dissenting view

As a member of the Barclay Committee, Professor Robert Pinker strongly disagreed with the notion of community social work. In a minority report of one he pointed to the problems of accountability with patch-based teams: what would be their relationship with senior management and elected members? He also lamented the Committee's strong criticism of social casework. Social work should practise what it knows how to do, he argued. He further argued that neighbourhood-based services were potentially invasive, with local residents ever aware that social workers would always have a presence throughout the neighbourhood.

He concluded that:

[it is] the prospect of the neighbourhood, or patch version of community social work which I find most disturbing. It conjures up the vision of a captainless crew under a patchwork ensign stitched together from remnants of the Red Flag and the Jolly Roger* – all with a licence and some with a

disposition to mutiny – heading in the gusty winds of populist rhetoric, with presumption as their figurehead and inexperience as their compass, straight for the reefs of public incredulity.

(Pinker 1982: 262)

*A reference to Roger Hadley, the foremost proponent of community social work at the time.

Discussion point

In regard to community social work, which of the positions set out in the above two boxes do you find yourself more in agreement with?

Cheshire social services department tries neighbourhood-based work

Following the Barclay Committee Report Cheshire County Council used 'areas of family stress', a precursor of the index of multiple deprivation produced by government, to apply for extra funding to build service resources on some of the disadvantaged council housing estates on the edge of Chester. The indicators aggregated the number of pupils receiving free school dinners, rates of family break-up, and the number of children coming into care. This did bring in some extra money that funded the appointment of community workers and allowed some early joint financing projects with the health service to get under way. In general, social work teams in Chester adapted some of the elements of community social work. But according to Craig Cawthorn, the district manager, at the time social workers' temporary focus on community was 'a bit of a fashion'. It could not ignore its own social control element even in that context. Yet particular neighbourhood based initiatives were successful – day nurseries that focused support and provided services for families with young children in ways that foreshadowed Sure Start (Cawthorn 2010).

Social work as maintenance

As social work retreated from its radical objectives as agents of change, the notion of maintenance as the prime social work task became more influential. Social workers, so maintenance theory argued, were not primarily engaged in social change; rather, their contribution was to sustain individual lives within existing social patterns. True, social work occupies an ambiguous position; it both performs social control functions and supports those who are not able to negotiate for themselves within the labour market. In that sense social work is inescapably a servant of the state. Among its responsibilities it engages in deviancy-controlling activities with individual clients. Even complex social problems are resolvable without root-and-branch restructuring of society; social work provided a means for channelling a modest level of benefits and services to those who need them most. In that sense social workers are inescapably part of the wider welfare state.

Martin Davies on maintenance

'In any society, there are bound to be yearnings for radical or revolutionary reform, but such feelings are not *in themselves* to be identified with social work. Political agitators or conflict theorists may regret this; they may think that the greater exposure of social workers to poverty and degradation should lead them to be activists in the front line of rebellion; and there may well be circumstances in one society or another which ultimately persuade social workers that their role as the maintenance mechanics of that society is no longer defensible or sustainable. But, unless or until that happens, it is a fundamental precept of the idea that social work is socially sanctioned (that is to say, created by, paid by and allowed to operate under the aegis of the existing regime) that its employees, *as social workers,* acknowledge a broad acceptance of the legitimacy of the government.'

Source: Davies 1981: 31.

Discussion point   Marxism or maintenance?

Reread the passages by Corrigan and Leonard on Marxism and social work at the beginning of this chapter and then the passage above by Martin Davies. Which perspective do you lean towards?

Maintenance as a function of social work called for a refocus on basic skills, such as interviewing, assessment and determining who the client is. It required capable written and verbal communication and professional standards in pursuit of publicly recognized objectives. It was also essential for the client to grasp the nature of social work. Among the important lessons of maintenance were:

- Handle the intake process with imagination, sensitivity and tact, putting client at ease.
- Be concerned with the client as a person and handle the personal in a professional manner.
- Identify client's expectations and relate these to the agency's obligations and resources.
- Be a good counsellor.

Social workers cannot deny that their role puts them in a position of power and privilege and they have to embrace the social control function – and see this as a contribution for the social system as a whole. Any potential for political change lies primarily in their relationship with their employer rather than their clients.

Anti-racism and anti-oppressive practice

In response to the riots in Brixton, south London, in the early 1980s the Scarman Report, while sensitive to the economic and social factors that would generate unrest, denied the existence of institutional racism and instead defined racism as a function of individual prejudice (Scarman 1982). In contrast to attitudes a decade later, the police themselves claimed that police 'misconduct' was overblown, a function of the street culture of black youth quick to exaggerate a grievance (Penketh 2000: 27).

By the mid-1980s, anti-racist perspectives – or at least 'race awareness' – pointed out the limitation of understanding racism in terms of individual prejudice and moved towards an analysis that saw racism inherent (or 'endemic in British society', in CCETSW's phrase of 1989 which it was subsequently forced to withdraw) in public attitudes and institutions. Studies of unemployment, youth justice and children in care pointed to the over-representation of minority ethnic groups, as did studies showing how black youths were more likely to be subject to stop and search by the police. Anti-racist strategies began to move beyond assimilationist and integrationist solutions. If racism was built into the structures and institutions of society, and these were underpinned by the state, then to uproot it effectively anti-racism required mobilization of coalitions within communities, workplaces and state institutions.

The Central Council for Education and Training in Social Work (CCETSW) by the late 1980s was developing its own strategy to move the entire social work profession, along with students being trained on CCETSW-approved courses, to the point of explicit commitment to anti-racist strategies. The Council offered a strategy in Paper 30 (CCETSW 1991) that stipulated that the curriculum for the new diploma in social work should include a strategy for tackling racism as an institutional phenomenon. It was a bold strategy which recognized that major institutions were structurally and institutionally racist, including the universities that delivered social work education and social work agencies themselves.

The question arises, why did CCETSW so strongly commit itself to an anti-racist strategy when the general political climate set by the Conservative government was generally antagonistic to such a stand? Penketh points to two reasons: first, the continuing legacy of radical social work, and second, the popular opposition to the government's domination of political culture, including its explicit attacks on gays and lesbians. But, Penketh argues, it was primarily the direct consequence of years of black students, black social workers and educators pressing forward with an anti-racist perspective (Penketh 2000: 52).

Institutional racism defined

Twenty years ago the concept of institutional racism, that is, racism built into the practices of organizations and agencies, was difficult for people to grasp. The idea that racism extended beyond individual prejudice and could be something that was unwittingly carried out, needed time to sink in. The paradox that racism was something that could happen in the conduct of agency personnel who were individually anti-racist in attitude was difficult to comprehend.

> The collective failure of an organization to provide an appropriate and professional service to people because of their colour, culture or ethnic origin. It can be seen or detected in processes, attitudes and behaviour which amount to discrimination through unwitting prejudice, ignorance, thoughtlessness and racist stereotyping which disadvantage minority ethnic people.
> (Macpherson 1999: para. 6.34)

Vigorous debate ensued over what was essentially a top-down strategy on the part of CCETSW. There were those on the political right – Professor Robert Pinker was one – who thought CCETSW should be stopped in its tracks (Pinker 1993). Others, on the left, thought that the CCETSW strategy often focused *only* on language, and as important as language was, it left aside the harder issues of how to tackle poverty and inequality (Webb 1991; Pierson 1999). Penketh (2000) noted the consequences of a top-down policy announced without adequate consultation: practice teachers received little preparatory training, social work education programmes that lagged behind faced the threat of de-validation, while debate over 'campus thought police' and other aspects of what much of the media identified as 'political correctness' played continuously in the press.

Despite limitations from the point of view of 2011, CCETSW's strategy was ahead of its time. It ran into difficulties and ridicule only because, in the early 1990s, institutional racism was a difficult and paradoxical concept to understand. Today such a policy would not be controversial.

Summary

- Radical social workers shunned social work's professional aspirations which they regarded as elitist and looked to the trade union movement to obtain higher salaries *and* to help reduce inequalities in wealth and power in society at large.

- Largely influenced by Marxism, radical social workers viewed society as dominated by social class and the conflict between classes, with social workers somewhat in between – a largely middle-class occupation but one entirely familiar with the struggles of those living below the poverty line.
- The social workers' strike of 1978–79 affected a relatively few local authorities – nor was it instigated by radicals but came about as individual branches of NALGO sought regrading and higher pay through local negotiations. But it did result in improvements in pay and conditions across the whole country.
- By the early 1980s the radicalism of the 1970s was in retreat, but left a legacy in the shape of community social work and anti-racist policies of CCETSW.
- Social work was in advance of other professions and occupations when CCETSW adopted anti-racist practice. It understood the nature of 'institutionalized racism' but met criticism for the top-down nature by which this policy was enforced.

Notes

1. I am grateful to John Webb for his detailed comments on the outcomes of the strike, which I draw on here.
2. The phrase 'social network' is now as likely to conjure up web-based contact among 'friends'; it is used here to refer to sustained face-to-face contact among family, friends and neighbours and other associational entities in a geographical community or community of interest.

Suggested reading

Bailey, R. and M. Brake (eds) (1975). *Radical Social Work*. London: Edward Arnold.
Barclay Committee (1982). *Social Workers: Their Role and Tasks*. London: Bedford Square Press.
Davies, M. (1981). *The Essential Social Worker: A Guide to Positive Practice*. London: Heinemann.

The papers of Margaret Thatcher are with the Thatcher Foundation at Churchill College, Cambridge, and are readily available on line.

9 Commissioning, Competences and 'Social Care'

Towards the end of the twentieth century, social work and social services departments worked in an environment very different from that which might have been comfortably predicted in 1975. This chapter covers the profound changes wrought from the 1990s onward. It examines:

- the introduction of market-like conditions and new public management into service provision;
- the trend to specialization in adult and children services;
- attempts to consolidate professional status by revamping training and regulatory systems from CCETSW to General Social Care Council to College of Social Work;
- the move towards personalization of services in the context of a hardening of welfare reform.

Social work and the marketplace

Britain itself changed rapidly through the 1980s. The argument continues, and may never be concluded, over whether on balance those changes freed up individual choice, aspiration and entrepreneurship or whether they produced selfishness and inequality. Both could be said to be true. By the late 1980s the Conservative government, having already brought market principles into council housing and other elements of the welfare state, was determined to do the same for social care.

Thus conflict between the objectives of the classic welfare state and the objectives of the market was brought out into the open. The classic welfare state had sought to 'de-commodify' people, that is, to ensure that people did not have to sell their labour power in the labour market in order to have a decent life and enjoy full citizenship, and to protect those unable to compete in the labour market for whatever reason – old age, incapacity, discrimination, caring responsibilities. Eventually welfare reform stood this proposition on its head, that participation in the labour market *is* the basis for citizenship and that welfare should assist in placing service users in work.

Many social work commentators and historians have noted that the organizational and functional culture of social work changed irretrievably with the passage of the NHS and Community Care Act 1990 (see Chapter 11). That Act reconfigured services on market-like principles on the back of which private sector management approaches became prominent (Lymbery 1998, 2001). This double impact upended social work values: relationships, counselling and support were blunted by an emphasis on assessment according to eligibility criteria. Standardization of procedures displaced the functions of counselling and support. Social workers' focus on the efficient use of their purchasing power had the unintended consequence of emphasizing risk management, dominating assessment of need and displacing preventive work altogether (Kemshall et al. 1997; Waterson 1999).

In what might be called the 'post-Seebohm' department (with de facto but not yet formal division between children and adult services), contending principles of normalization and specialization underlay the move towards community care. As for judgements around provision of care services after the 1993 implementation of the NHS and Community Care Act, the power of professional judgement to make choices among different courses of action clashed with more elaborate systems of categorizing clients for eligibility. This tension lay at the heart of the reorganized personal social services of the 1990s. Stripping social services departments of their service provider role served to disperse the capacities of their once functional unity by reducing their role to specifying and awarding contract. In retaining overall control of local authority budgets, it was effectively central government that remained the key actor in the contract culture.

Discussion point How should the social worker have responded?

A community psychiatric nurse telephones the team to ask for an assessment of one of her patients to see what services that person might need. The social worker asks what services the patient needed. The nurse says she is not sure but thought that that was the social worker's job to determine. The social worker asks impatiently what the nurse meant by assessment – a home care assessment, day care assessment or hospital assessment? The nurse was not sure but wanted the social worker to visit the patient to find out. The social worker decided the patient needed a 'home care assessment' over the telephone and passed the referral over to the home care team manager.

How should the social worker have responded to the community psychiatric nurse?

New public management

The introduction of care management principles brought professional discretion under managerial control by converting spenders into budget managers. In the years of the classic welfare state, public sector services were built on firm procedural rules governing the way they should work and with an ethos that was, in those services' own perception, dedicated to the public good. The tenets of new public management challenged that ethos:

- Budgets became transparent in accounting terms, with costs linked to what services actually did and those outputs measured by quantitative performance indicators.
- Quasi-market negotiations and distinctions between purchaser and provider replaced previously unified structures that planned *and* provided public services.
- The injection of greater plurality into service provision – drawing on public and independent sector organizations – allowed users more scope to 'exit', that is, simply decline to use the services of a particular provider, as opposed to relying on 'voice', that is, building up political pressure on large-scale public providers.
- Most importantly, setting up cost centres inside public services affected collaborations within and among organizations, with their becoming a chain of low-trust relationships between agents rather than a collaboration among trustees and beneficiaries of the public good (Dunleavy and Hood 1994: 9).

Accounts of this transition to the post-Seebohm department are uniformly negative (Dominelli 1996; Jones 2001; Harris 2003; Rogowski 2010). They variously describe as a 'neo-liberal project' the organizational culture in which:

- managers told social workers *not* to form relationships as contact with users was fleeting;
- front-line workers were kept out of meetings at which resources were decided;
- the division between front-line workers and managers only widened (Jones 2001: 552).

From educators to practitioners, from academic journal articles to issues of *Community Care*, there was regular testimony that social work had become more office based, with less direct work with users, that organizational change was continuous but never based on consultation with those who delivered the services. Rough estimates suggested that whereas in the early 1990s the requirements of the bureaucracy took up 30 per cent of the social worker's week, for a care manager in the late 1990s and early 2000s that figure had risen to 90 per cent.

Gains for users

It can be argued that in the 1990s individual users started to gain more control over decisions that affected them. The Disabled Persons (Services, Consultation and Representation) Act 1986 had already charged the local authority with the duty to assess a disabled person's needs under the Chronically Sick and Disabled Persons Act 1970 (CSDP Act) when requested to do so. The Carer's Recognition and Services Act 1995 obliged the local authority to assess carers' needs while it carried out an assessment under the NHS and Community Care Act, the Children Act 1989 or the CSDP Act. The Community Care (Direct Payments) Act 1996 permitted individual users to receive funding directly from the local authority to purchase the services they thought they needed rather than have the local authority fund those services. Originally only for people with disability under 65 years old, the arrangement was progressively expanded; the Health and Social Care Act 2001 finally made it a duty for local authorities to provide direct payments for all those eligible over the age of 16.

Thus the first steps towards individual control and personalization (see Chapter 11) were under way, albeit slowly. More importantly, within social work thinking itself service users were accorded greater influence and user participation in decisions became a critical component of social work decision making (Braye and Preston-Shoot 1995; Braye 2000).

The White Paper *Our Health, Our Care, Our Say* (Department of Health 2006) placed the user at the centre of the system of obtaining care – always with the proviso that that system operated in conditions of scarcity constraining the user choices from the start. It completed the revolution begun twenty years previously by the Griffiths Report, by separating fully the role of assessment and commissioning of services from service provision. Commissioners were made accountable to users and able to draw on a wider range of community services, not just health or social care. The White Paper also suggested creating independent advocates to help users make informed choices. Users as individual budget holders was the logical end point – empowering them to make their own care choices.

Choice, however, proved a difficult terrain for users since it involved navigating systems with which they were unfamiliar and where they were uncertain what their money was buying. Despite this apparent step forward, evidence from the late 1990s and early 2000s indicates that organizational policy and professional power continued to shape assessment process in particular directions, with social worker discretionary decisions playing an important part (Rummery and Glendinning 1999; Postle 2001). There is evidence, however, that social work adapts and persists in shaping its tasks as it understands those tasks even in organizational and procedural environments that are contrary to its longstanding values (Jordan 2004; Lloyd 2006: 1180; Cawthorn 2010). Professional ideology – linking notions of fairness with meticulous attention to eligibility criteria while at the same believing fully in the autonomy of the individual user – proved a potent force, and professional interactions with users actually shaped the developing service (Sullivan 2009).

UPIAS statement 1975

'[The] alternative struggle proposed by the Union is logically developed from a social theory of disability. We pose the question as to why the Alliance and its "experts" have not produced an adequate social theory of disability. We ourselves look for our expertise to the wealth of talent and intellectual imagination of disabled people, which will be freed for expression once we contemplate our own situation from our own collective experience. The Union therefore seeks to help disabled people to recognise and oppose all approaches which can only see answers to our problems in terms of different forms of charity. We call on physically impaired people and others who want to help to join the Union and help us build a mass, democratic organisation, with a principled approach to disability that will struggle to win the right to employment in integrated work situations, and to eliminate from our society the disablement of people who have physical impairments.'

Source: Finkelstein 1975: 9.

Throughout the 1990s and into the twenty-first century there was continuous discussion of whether social work could 'empower' users and, if so, how. This issue has still not been disentangled. It can, for instance, be argued that in terms of moral argument influence was the other way round: that advocacy and self-advocacy groups taught social work convincing lessons about users' needs and, more important, about the oppressions and discriminations particular user groups faced.

Forceful messages came from several different directions. People with physical disability and organizations representing them offer one powerful example. The declaration of the Union of the Physically Impaired Against Segregation (UPIAS) in 1975 can stand in as the start point for the social model of disability now widely adopted by social work. That statement not only rejects paternalist and medical models of disability but lashes into those who were campaigning for higher state benefits. Both had failed in the eyes of UPIAS because they had not touched the core problems facing people with disability.

The social disability model gained wide traction within social work through the work of Michael Oliver who first used the phrase in the early 1980s. Over the next decade it was extended to cover those with learning disability as well. Broadly, the model reversed the interpretation of disability – rather than an individual tragedy or condition requiring charity (or benefits), it was society's constricted view of impairments that so constrained the movements of and opportunities for disabled people. The model required root and branch reform of social attitudes and social infrastructure – from pavements and transportation to education and labour market reform.

Discussion point   Would you turn back the clock?

Given the profound changes which care management and new public management techniques introduced to social work services, if you could, would you turn back the clock to a time *before* that? To help you decide, draw up a balance sheet of what was lost and what was gained by the introduction of quasi-markets in social care. If you decide that you would prefer to work at time before 1990, what period would you choose?

The advocacy and self-advocacy movement

Other rights-based advocacy organizations also helped to educate social work and social workers throughout the 1980s and 1990s. The National Association of Young People in Care (now the Youth Parliament) and the Children's Legal Centre, among others, promoted children's rights that again took some twenty years to become a force that shaped social work and the broader legal landscape. In 1987 Mike Lindsay became the first children's rights officer to be appointed by a local authority, for some years the only one. By the late 1990s children's advocacy organizations had grown in size and number, mostly in the voluntary sector – Barnardo's, Children's Rights Alliance for England, Who Cares? Trust, National Youth Advocacy Service – and in 2004 recognition by government came with the creation of a Children's Commissioner for England in the Children Act 2004 and statements that the children's voice should be at the centre of their time in care.

A similar pathway was trodden within mental health. The National Institute of Mental Health moved from a long-established charity to campaigning and advocacy roles as first MIND (the National Association of Mental Health changed its name to MIND in 1972), SANE (formed in 1986) and a myriad of mental health survivors groups applied pressure to humanize, localize and recognize the rights of those suffering from mental health problems.

The pathways of influence of advocacy, and especially self-advocacy, groups on social work require further investigation. From a profession-centric point of view it may seem that social work itself developed strategies of empowerment. However, from outside the profession the fact that external groups were the motors for expanding notions of citizenship urging participation in key decision-making, developing models that upended a hundred years and more of social work practice, seems beyond doubt.

Reforming professional qualifications

Historically there were two essential elements through which social work sought to establish its professional status: the first was a fully fledged three-year university-based degree for qualification to be followed by systematic post-qualifying training; the second, a system of registration. By the mid-1980s the Conservative government resisted any changes to the level of qualification needed for social work. Against this headwind CCETSW lobbied hard for a degree-level qualification through much of the 1980s. A review of social work education commissioned by government in 1984 finally led to the introduction of a single qualification, the Diploma in Social Work, in 1988. The 'DipSW' brought to an end the twin-track training programme – Certificate of Qualification in Social Work (CQSW) for social workers and the Certificate in Social Service (CSS) for non social workers in social services departments, such as social work assistants and managers of care homes, established in 1977. The new central role for employers, which had not been part of the CQSW programmes, gave rise to some concern among university social work educationists that this would constrict the curriculum and reduce the element of critical analysis of policy and practice. The DipSW ceased to be an entry route for probation officers in England and Wales in the mid-1990s (but remained so for Scotland and Northern Ireland), as probation became more closely linked with the prison service under the control of the Home Office.

The review of the CQSW had found that social work training required a minimum of three years' study, leading some to hope, even to expect, that government would fund the social work degree for which CCETSW had been lobbying so hard. The eventual rejection of this recommendation was both an indicator that social work's standing with government was not high and also a profound rejection of professional aspiration.[1] As a leading director said at the time, government opting for a two-year diploma was 'an eloquent testimony of the continued failure of social work, its professional bodies and its practitioners to define what differentiates social work from other forms of intervention' (Bamford 1990: 71, quoted in Orme 2001: 614).

As we noted in the previous chapter, social work itself was ambivalent about how far to extend its formal status of profession and whether to include or exclude those without social work qualification from its ranks. The DipSW did move beyond this impasse. It was offered at non-graduate, graduate and postgraduate level and therefore could be taken over two, three or four years. It also allowed the development of 'pathways', enabling students to develop some specialization. Some departments applied its principle of unifying the two major qualifications retrospectively by developing part-time, university-based courses for those of its staff with the CSS qualification to be trained in areas – particularly the law – that would bring them level with the requirements of the new DipSW.

Following election of the Labour government in 1997, consultants were brought in to re-examine the issue of qualifying training and whether or not social workers were required to be qualified (see box below). On the basis of the consultants' report the White Paper *Quality Strategy for Social Care* (Department of Health 2000b) now referred to 'social care', of which social work was only a part. To ensure quality of service it moved away from a focus on a social work framework and instead looked to workforce planning and a new organization, the Social Care Institute of Excellence. Emphasis now rested on users' experiences of the service and not on who delivers it (Orme 2001). There was no attempt to define social work other than to note its 'emphasis on rights, responsibilities, citizenship and participation' and to link these with skills such as 'assessment, so that decision making and care planning are based on a sound analysis and understanding of the person's unique personality, history and circumstances' (Department of Health 2000b: 37). Crucially, however, the White Paper called for a three-year degree course to train social workers.

JM Consulting reviews social work training

'Social Work is an emerging discipline. It does not have all the attributes of the more established professions, but we believe that it can and should have similar aims in terms of excellence of practice; an ethos of service to clients and the public; an evidence/research base for action; and the ability and will to create and operate to a regime of high standards and continual improvement. We are certain that the public expect this. The key element of this is that it places a responsibility on individual social workers to be accountable for their practice and for their own continuing professional development.'

Source: JM Consulting 1999: 4.

The consultants rejected the notion that social workers operated within a predetermined framework of procedures and were not required to exercise independent judgement, with the implication that employers or managers who determine procedures are primarily accountable for their performance. They noted that social workers have to:

- make complex assessments on behalf of clients (involving personal health, family circumstances, financial problems and housing/ environmental factors);
- support clients in making their own decisions;
- gain client ownership of intervention strategies;
- make critical decisions regarding client safety or loss of liberty in mental health and child protection which require mature and independent judgement;
- work alongside other professionals in multi-professional and multi-agency teams and need to be able to work on behalf of their clients from a position of equal confidence and esteem.

General social work council

The idea of a general social work council overseeing a register of qualified social workers was first proposed in 1977. As the more fractious 1980s wore on, with public attention called to social workers' failures, doubts surfaced about professional competence. Those opposed to the idea of a professional body regulating social work – whether in government or within social work – argued that a council would invariably lead to a sense of specialist status that would distance social workers from both colleagues they had to work closely with in residential, day and domiciliary services, and the users they worked with. In short they would lose the 'democratic quotient' that came with *not* being a recognized profession with a certain status attached.

The mixed economy of care arising in the wake of the NHS and Community Care Act 1990 spawned a range of providers from different backgrounds attempting to achieve particular standards – hence government began to view regulation in general as a tool to achieve better standards rather than as a means of professional self-regulation. Social work in particular was ripe for regulation after the murder of Victoria Climbié, a child with whom social workers were involved. The Care Standards Act 2000 took the step to establish the General Social Care Council, with powers to maintain a register of qualified social workers, and to strike practitioners from that register. It was also given a remit to develop the entire social care sector, particularly to assist in workforce planning. Crucially, it was also given oversight of social work training (with CCETSW then abolished).

Three parallel bodies were established in the other parts of the United Kingdom: the Scottish Social Services Council, the Care Council for Wales and the Northern Ireland Social Care Council. Altogether the four national councils were driven by the plurality of social care service, including voluntary and for-profit sectors, to standardize practice and ensure application of values across all delivery. While Wales had its own Care Council, registration of staff to work with adults was to be kept by the Secretary of State at Westminster. The Scottish Social Services Council took on all regulatory tasks under the authority of the Scottish government. The Northern Ireland Social Care Council's remit was similar to that of the General Social Care Council (GSCC) for England.

The GSCC for England was set up in October 2001 and registration of all social workers, social work students and social care staff began in 2003 confirming their fitness to practice. This broad remit was far wider than that anticipated by those who had argued for a professional register – it was envisaged that some one million social care workers would enrol. From the outset it was plain that the GSCC was never going to function as a coherent source of professionalism nor provide a guarantee of a fully qualified workforce.

The General Social Care Council

'The draft standards just issued by the council include duties on workers to strive for and maintain the trust and confidence of service users; to take responsibility for their own practice and learning; not to abuse, exploit or harm users, colleagues or carers; and to inform their employer about any physical, mental or legal difficulties that might affect their performance.

'The Care Standards Act specifies several categories of staff who will be required to register. These include social workers; staff in children's homes; care homes; residential family centres; domiciliary care; fostering agencies or voluntary adoption agencies, and all those who manage these staff. Regulations may also require registration of any other staff involved in delivering personal care, inspecting children's homes, independent schools and colleges, those employed in day centres and trainee social workers.'

Source: Batty 2002.

There was strong objection to the continuity between the Conservative government policy in relation to skills training and that of the Labour government which replaced it in 1997. As one cogent observer stated: 'the one arm of social work which had achieved a fully qualified workforce was moving to a differentiated workforce with low levels of qualification' (Orme 2001: 617). The licensed national Training Organization for Personal Social Services (TOPSS) defined occupational standards while the GSCC validated the training, and universities and colleges delivered it. In fact, TOPSS was forced to pay far more attention to the vast unqualified workforce, developing standards and pathways based on the National Vocational Qualification (NVQ) framework introduced as far back as 1986. The concern was that some social work tasks would be downgraded to the level of technical knowledge; on the other hand, training was extended and career pathways opened up to a social care workforce, mostly women, that had previously largely been ignored. Thus in the early 2000s what social work had considered its own historic province – professional registration – was being mixed in with other occupational groups, standards and training pathways. Boundaries were blurring, job titles changing and, beyond that, tasks which were once the province of skilled social workers were now to be found in a raft of new kinds of posts: Connexions personal advisers, back to work advisers, intensive family support casework.

Burial of the generic team (the generic worker had been lost years before), a process that had been under way for a dozen years or more, became inevitable. Tasks were now to be defined user group by user group, for example by modes of practice in child protection, mental health, safeguarding older people, and care mangement and so on. The assumption behind this was that what once were regarded as the preserve of social workers could now be undertaken by a vocationally qualified social care workforce, a direction 'at odds with a quality strategy that asserts the complexity and significance of the work and demands training and regulation' (Orme 2001: 621). Orme's prognosis was: 'It seems likely that the majority of the workforce will be trained only to the level of the tasks in which they are engaged, as identified in occupational standards' (ibid.).

The Social Work Task Force and Social Work Reform Board

The division of social work activities – children and families in one organization ultimately responsible to the Department of Education and adult services responsible to the Department of Health – marked the formal end of the generic department. Social work developments that arose from the creation of two new state agencies are discussed in the following two chapters. Two of the hoped for outcomes, however, that the division of services failed to bring about were (i) clarity to what it is that social work does, and (ii) clearer ideas about the composition and direction of the workforce.

Within a short time a Social Work Task Force (SWTF) was commissioned by government to bring some coherent vision to the future of social work. The suggestions of the Task Force could have been written in any of the previous five decades: better training, better working conditions, stronger leadership, regular supply of confident, adaptable professionals. It also sought to develop greater understanding from the public, service users and government itself about the role and purpose of social work.

The Task Force offered a number of recommendations:

- the creation of a national college;
- all social work students should complete a first probationary year after finishing their course and should not be considered qualified until that year is completed;
- clear, universal and binding standards for employers, including supervision;
- publish performance on caseload ceilings and other controls;
- establish a national framework for career structure and career development, including an MA in social work;
- introduce licence to practise;
- undertake a programme of action on public understanding, with colleges playing a leading role;
- a board to oversee the reform programme.

The SWTF defines social work

As one of its aims the SWTF sought to increase public awareness of what social work does. To help achieve this it provided an explanation to the public – what it called a 'public description' – of what social work does. It read:

> Social work helps adults and children to be safe so they can cope and take control of their lives again. Social workers make life better for people in crisis who are struggling to cope, feel alone and cannot sort out their problems unaided.
>
> How social workers do this depends on the circumstances. Usually they work in partnership with the people they are supporting – check out what they need, find what will help them, build their confidence, and open doors to other services. Sometimes, in extreme situations such as where people are at risk of harm or in danger of hurting others, social workers have to take stronger action – and they have the legal powers and duties to do this.
>
> You may think you already do this for your friends and family but social workers have specialist training in fully analysing problems and unmet needs, in how people develop and relate to each other, in understanding the challenging circumstances some people face, and in how best to help them cope and make progress. They are qualified to tell when people are in danger of being harmed or harming others and know when and how to use their legal powers and responsibilities in these situations.
>
> You may think that you'll never need a social worker but there is a wide range of situations where you or your family might need one, such as

caring for family members
having problems with family relationships and conflict
struggling with challenges of growing old
suffering serious personal troubles and mental distress
having drug and alcohol problems
facing difficulties as a result of disability
being isolated within the community
having practical problems with money or housing

(Social Work Task Force 2009: 67)

In the same document, the Task Force also set out its ambitions for reform:

As reform unfolds and conditions improve, social work needs to become a profession which takes responsibility for the quality of its practice. It should use the best evidence to determine how it can be most effective. It should be respected and supported, but held fairly to account by Government, employers, educators, regulators and the public.

(ibid.: 6)

Discussion point   How effective is the SWTF's definition with the public?

Read carefully the SWTF's public definition of social work in the box above. What are its strengths? How useful do you find it in explaining social work to non-social-work friends? What are its shortcomings?

The 'core' of social work is smaller than twenty years ago: ancillary and para-social workers shoulder a greater part of the work, private agency staff are utilized in great numbers, social work tasks, such as adoption and foster home finders, are hived off to voluntary organizations. With the spread of individual budgets the social work role centres more around care management while support and monitoring passes to voluntary organizations (Cawthorn 2011). The Reform Board is now in place at the time of writing. The difficulty of pinning down what social workers do remains. The former Children, Schools and Families select committee and the Social Work Reform Board both noted that social work standards are confusing and the Board is intent on clarifying those standards within an overarching capabilities framework – to set new standards for entry level as well as set standards for education and training.

Coalition attitudes towards social work

The coalition government's policies for social work transfers the GSCC's functions to the Health and Care Professions Council in England, a regulatory body covering some 300,000 varying professionals (the GSCC was responsible for one-third that number). Responsibilities for registration of social workers are devolved to Scotland, Wales and Northern Ireland, with only England remaining under the control of Westminster although a link will continue among the four national councils to permit cross-registration.

The Social Work Reform Board aligns itself with the 'big society'

In a recent set of minutes the Social Work Reform Board aligned itself with concepts behind the 'big society'. It noted that it is

> enormously encouraged by the commitment given by this government to implementing the Task Force's recommendations. The government's vision is of a society in which individuals feel both free and powerful enough to help themselves and their own communities. Social workers have a significant role to play in protecting the children, adults and families they work with and empowering them to make positive changes in their lives. The government wants to reduce the bureaucracy and burdens faced by organisations and communities. It has said that in order to bring about change and improve social work services, the sector should be empowered to shape and embed reforms that address the needs of local communities without excessive central prescription and regulation.
>
> In November 2010, the government published its vision for adult social care. This recognises the important role of social workers in supporting and protecting adults while empowering them to make their own decisions about shaping and buying services tailored to their needs. The trialing of Social Work Practices and the potential for mutuals and cooperatives in social care means that the settings in which social workers practise and are employed may change significantly over time.
>
> (Social Work Reform Board 2011)

Summary

- On the recommendations of the Griffiths Report the Conservative government introduced market reforms into social care at the end of the 1980s based chiefly on the principle of separating purchasers of services from the providers of those services. In this new context local authorities were to be come 'enablers' and not primarily providers.

- Some aspects of private sector management were brought into public services – dubbed 'managerialist' by critics or 'new public management'.
- Arguments and pressure from user advocacy and self-advocacy groups substantially changed social work practice by the 1990s.
- By the early 2000s social work acquired some of the attributes of a profession which it had long sought: a three-year degree for qualification and a general council. However, both had to establish credibility as questions over the definition of social work remained among the public and government. The current negotiations around a college of social work and its relationship to the coalition government are still unfolding.

Note

1. The author well recalls the sense of dismay inside the departmental training team where he worked when word came out that government had rejected three-year training in favour of a two-year diploma. We had confidently expected one thing and got quite another.

Suggested reading

Harris, J. (2003). *The Social Work Business*. London: Routledge.
Rogowski, S. (2010). *Social Work: The Rise and Fall of a Profession?* Bristol: Policy Press.

10 Social Work with Children and Young People

This chapter charts the pivotal developments in children's services as additional statutory responsibilities, the force of public opinion and heightened awareness of risk all intersected to bring a new intensity and responsibility to social work. It covers:

- the children's service that emerged in the wake of the Second World War;
- the changes in law and practice concerning young offenders;
- the renewed focus on child abuse;
- the major reforms embodied in the Children Act 1989;
- the creation of children's services established by Every Child Matters.

Separation and the emotional needs of children

The evacuation of children in the early years of the Second World War (see Chapter 7) prompted an urgent national debate about fostering and tilted public opinion towards greater local authority involvement in the process. The number of social workers focusing on child care also greatly increased during the war. Building on the voluntary work of the care committees, their salaried organizers, and social workers attached to the education departments of local authorities the outlines of a children's social work service began to emerge. A spotlight was also shone on residential regimes and the staff skills for looking after children while in care (Holman 1996). A consensus emerged that children should not be left under the care of the public assistance committee of local authorities because of their close association with the stigma of the Poor Law. By 1943 informal committees had been set up within government to consider the plight of children left homeless as a result of the war and to examine arrangements for a children's service in light of the recommendations of the Beveridge Report. The Ministry of Health in particular looked forward to the final break-up of the Poor Law and the consolidation of all services for children in need within 'a single, well-qualified and sympathetic administration' (Holman 1996: 7; Ministry of Health 1943).

The experiences of children separated from their parents

John Bowlby (1907–1990), a psychiatrist and psychologist working at the Tavistock Institute, developed his concepts of attachment, maternal deprivation and loss from his studies of children at this time. Before the war Bowlby was one of several psychoanalysts in Britain who argued that there was a 'repression of tenderness' and that children should be provided with emotional education in order to have a prosperous and harmonious society. Bowlby was a confirmed social democrat and a strong supporter of the newly created welfare state, believing that love and social responsibility had to be enabled in the development of the individual personality.

Bowlby had an able collaborator in Mary Ainsworth (1913–1999) who published her own studies and broadened the notion of attachment to care givers rather than just mothers. Together the two researchers exerted huge influence on social work practice with children throughout the second half of the twentieth century, affecting, in particular, assessments of child–parent relationships and decisions around whether children should be placed for long-term fostering or adoption.

The death of Dennis O'Neill

While the consensus among social workers and government circles pointed to a new social work service for children based in local authorities, the death of a child in foster care gave the discussions added urgency. Dennis O'Neill had been evacuated in 1939, separated from his two brothers and placed with foster parents at Bank Farm in Minsterly, Shropshire. In January 1945 he was beaten on the chest with a stick by his foster parents and died of cardiac arrest.

The ensuing enquiry did not have to look far for causes. The report, known as the Monckton Report after the chairperson of the enquiry, concluded that a number of factors lay behind Dennis's death: untrained staff, inadequate supervision, fragmented services. While government had already announced its intention to establish a wide-ranging committee to restructure state-provided child care services, the fate of Dennis O'Neill focused public opinion on the issues of child care and created a climate in which politicians felt compelled to act (Monckton 1945).

Developments leading to the Children Act 1948

Public opinion, galvanized by the war, was already engaged and played a forceful role in reconstructing children's services. Margery Allen (1897–1976) led a vigorous national campaign to provide better care for children that broke with Poor Law attitudes once and for all. In response, the wartime coalition government set up a committee of enquiry in March 1945 with a civil servant, Myra Curtis, as chairperson and several members who were either social workers or who had experience in child care. The committee's report – the Curtis Report – was delivered in 1946 and gave a lengthy account of the conditions and kinds of services that prevailed before the war. Indeed, two-thirds of the report was devoted to exposing the terrible conditions that children in public care, particularly within workhouses, were brought up in and noted that nearly 33,000 children were still in buildings governed by Poor Law regulations (Curtis 1946).

The Committee's strategic aim was to bring sympathy, attentiveness and individual care to a newly formed children's service in which the state, as corporate parent, would look after the needs of children in care. It recommended that this new service be based in local authorities which should appoint highly qualified children's officers to lead the new service. It also declared that the local authority should make every effort to keep a child within the family but, failing that, should foster children who retained some ties with their parents. Curtis also suggested that when local authorities assumed parental rights under the Children Act 1933, that should not be simply achieved by a committee resolution but involve court-appointed guardians representing the interests of the child.

In Scotland the Clyde Report (Clyde 1946) had already anticipated many of the Curtis recommendations. Set up at the same time, it reported first, in July 1946, and called attention to the fragmented responsibility of children's services, the hard conditions in which children were kept both in Poor Law institutions and in the large soulless children's homes run by voluntary organizations, and the lack of regular visits to foster homes. As did Curtis, the Clyde Report recommended that all services to do with children, then currently spread out over many different bodies, be unified under a single local authority committee.

The Children Act 1948 reflected many of the Curtis recommendations and was passed with support across the political spectrum. The Labour government of the time, with its large majority, fully supported the principle that local authorities would bring 'warmth and humanity', as the Minister of Health, Aneurin Bevan (1897–1960) put it, to caring for children in need. Under the Act, local authorities were to provide for children whose parents could not look after them through new children's departments under a qualified children's officer. The Act also empowered the local authority to pay for the further education and training of children in their care – a radically different ethos from past practice which had required authorities to 'set to work' orphans and destitute children and gave the authorities powers to inspect and register children's homes in their area.

The Act also required local authorities to restore those children received into care (that is, with the parents' agreement) to their natural home if appropriate. Although we now regard this as a standard duty, at the time it marked a break with the past in that Poor Law authorities and later the public assistance committees of the local authorities had no such duty placed on them – nor did they have the expertise or case records to effect a return home had they wanted to (Heywood 1978: 156).

This new duty underscored the need for skilled casework to work towards returning individual children to their families and to dealing with problematic parents. Social work was no longer concerned only with removing children from their environment or viewing reception into care as an irrevocable step after which a permanent substitute home had to be found, as it had been in the past. Maintaining some link with natural parents, paying fares for instance so that parents could visit children placed some distance from their home, became one of the social worker's chief tasks. As Heywood observed 'From this changed approach, building on and preserving what is good within the family, however weak and unsatisfactory, it became possible to see the problem of the deprived child and the failing parents as an interrelated whole' (Heywood 1978: 158).

Children's departments: ethos and practice

The Children Act 1948 marked a great leap forward in promoting expertise in working with families and is a significant mark in the professionalizing of social work. Although children's departments were relatively small they embodied a progressive and optimistic spirit that drew many social workers into its ranks. The Association of Child Care Officers (ACCO), formed in 1949, quickly became one of the most influential social work professional organizations, one that not only cultivated ties with government and members of Parliament but also grew accustomed to looking more widely at the origins of a family's problems. These characteristics would prove useful in the debate around preventive work and in promoting the recommendations of the Seebohm Committee in the 1960s.

The professional framework adopted by child care officers in the 1950s was ostensibly psychodynamic or 'psychosocial' in orientation (see Chapter 7) tempered by pragmatism. Casework was a framework not an ideology. While it emphasized analysing relationships within the family, it also provided a source of professional confidence and a starting point for understanding families and the relationship between parents and children that was not otherwise available (Craig Cawthorn 2010).

While the Act placed faith in social work expertise, the legal system within which that expertise operated harked back to an earlier time, creating a disjunction between social work and legal solutions to meeting children's needs. Adoption, for example, was regarded by the judicial system as a matter of legal status rather than as a way of providing for children in need. And despite Adoption Acts in 1949 and 1958, adoption law 'travelling in a compartment of its own marked "legal status" ', as Stephen Cretney put it (Cretney 2004: 684), remained under the jurisdiction of the Lord Chancellor and not the Ministry of Health that had oversight of work with children.

There was conflict too in removing children compulsorily from families. The grounds for doing so still lay with the Children and Young Persons Act 1933 which required that unnecessary suffering or injury to health be established – there was no provision on which assistance, whether financial or through family support work, could be given to parents having difficulties in looking after their children. The Children Act 1948 also did not provide that power, although forms of family support – provision of material aid, domestic help, guidance in home management, parental understanding of child development, as well as initiatives such as residential care for whole families and intensive family casework – had all been part of the discussions before the Act had been passed (Packman 1975: 53).

'Humanizing' children's homes, as Bob Holman (1996) has put it, was a first step after the creation of children's departments in 1948 which in essence involved breaking up the old large institutions to create family group homes of not more than twelve children. To approximate family life, each home was overseen by a married couple, with the husband going out to work – a model favoured in both England and Scotland (Brill and Thomas 1964; Holman 1996).

Such moves could not and did not happen overnight given the weight of history. In Manchester, for example, there were 886 children in eight large, local authority residential homes and 286 in voluntary homes. These establishments had previously been under the wing of the education, social welfare and health departments of the local authority, embracing a range of functions – 'receiving homes' (for those being received into care), separate remand homes for girls and boys, an approved school and clusters of cottage homes, homes for boys aged 8–15 'unsuitable for boarding out', and, in Manchester, a large residential nursery for 100 children (Holman 1996: 17).

Developing the case for preventive work

Following the passage of the Children Act 1948, and through the 1950s, child care social workers looked for greater flexibility, and began developing the case for greater powers to deal with neglect and to work with families to prevent the need to take children into care or to help with reunification following removal of a child. 'Boarding out officers', their official designation reflecting their key task of the removal and placement of children, gradually became child care officers, reflecting a more diverse set of objectives. (The Curtis Committee had recommended case loads of between 100 and 150 for each officer.) Early on, practitioners saw the limits of boarding-out work and began to see that preventing a child's coming into care should be a major element of their work.

Child care officers recognized the value of preventive work and engaged in intensive casework with specific families which combined frequent visiting with practical advice and material aid as well as persuasion and direct instruction. It was deemed important to build relationships with the children involved so that, should they be removed, it would be by people they knew (Packman 1975: 58). The officers began to examine existing links with relatives and neighbours as potential sources of care for children – acknowledging that fostering a child with people the child knew was less distressing for the child.

Homelessness proved a major reason for children coming into care through the 1950s – in some authorities the proportion was as high as 20 per cent. Material deprivation and lack of community spirit occasionally prompted the appointment of a child care worker living on a housing estate with the aim to foster community spirit and to draw child care officers into the life of the estate through joint outings.

Tom White's recollection

Tom White, later director of social services in Coventry and later still chief executive of the National Children's Home, began his social work career as a child care officer in north Devon in 1957. He recounts in his autobiography:

> When on my first morning I was allocated a caseload of 80+ adolescent boys plus a pile of other miscellaneous enquiries, I realised, much as I didn't like the idea, I'd have to protest immediately. . .
>
> I felt strongly about the development of social work as a profession. There was a common attitude among Councillors and the public (if they thought about it) that as the vast majority of families brought up children satisfactorily that Children's Departments could be staffed by anyone who had a bit of common sense and a good family life. But that was to completely misunderstand the task – dealing with seriously deprived and disturbed children was *not* like bringing up your own and a significant proportion of the children we dealt with were in that category. Increasingly research, much of which was based on the experience of the placement of evacuees in the war, together with studies of children in institutions etc. had demonstrated the complexity of the task – the Curtis Committee had been clear in recommending the creation of a new trained, skilled profession to deal with deprived children.
>
> (White 2011)

By the late 1950s ACCO began to exert pressure to provide a legal basis for preventive work. Such lobbying particularly took advantage of an issue that had become pressing for politicians: the rise in youth offending rates.

The Ingleby Committee in its report of 1960 examined policies towards young offenders and whether local authorities should be given powers to prevent child neglect, seen as a major cause of youth offending (Ingleby 1960).

The subsequent Children and Young Persons Act 1963 placed on local authorities the duty to diminish 'the need to receive children into or keep them in care' by making available advice, guidance and assistance 'as may promote the welfare of children'. It could do so through any provisions the local authorities thought fit, including 'giving assistance in kind or, in exceptional circumstances, in cash'. Hence the tag 'Section 1 money' was born – familiar to a generation of social workers – and recycled with exactly the same wording in section 1 of the Child Care Act 1980.

There were consequences, foreseen and unforeseen, of formalizing this power in law. A raft of small-scale but imaginative initiatives developed across the country: family advice centres in some cities, mobile foster mothers, who went to live with families in Cornwall, friendship clubs for isolated mothers, parent training for mothers having difficulties in child rearing or house management, appointment of village representatives to respond to emergencies, the drawing up of lists of sympathetic landlords (Packman 1975: 70).

More slowly, section 1 of the Act also created the perception that children's departments had a social security role and in particular had become an agent for debt relief – especially utility bills. This was not just in the eyes of users who sought relief but also in the eyes of other public agencies, such as the then nationalized gas and electricity companies which saw a way to clear debts on their books that were beyond the resources of debtor families themselves. This capacity to meet material need with cash proved a double-edged sword, intertwining debt relief with the capacity of the family to achieve specific goals. Thus, although unforeseen in the campaign for preventive powers, the 'coercive social worker' appeared at least in academic literature (Handler 1973), that is, the practitioner who could threaten to withhold cash support. This was a new tool with ambiguous consequences: the social worker now was able to dangle powerful carrots in front of families as long as they did what the social worker requested – and conversely withdraw cash assistance if there was low compliance.

Barbara Kahan, children's officer in Oxfordshire

Barbara Kahan (1920–2000) was appointed children's officer for Oxfordshire children's department in 1950, and began work in a department with one room and one employee – herself – and a stack of public assistance files. After six weeks she was able to hire a young secretary. Kahan had a caseload of her own as well as managed the department as it grew. In the years that followed she became the prime exponent of preventive work for which Oxfordshire was nationally recognized. As an early proponent of 'coordination' – partnership working as we would now call it – she enlisted other agencies to tackle child welfare needs and developed ways of channelling support, material and otherwise, to families at the end of their tether. Shortly following the passage of the Children and Young Persons Act 1963 some 655 children and their families were being assisted, with nine new referrals every week (Packman 1975: 68). By the middle of 1965, child care officers in Oxfordshire were supervising 700 children in their homes – a greater number than were in the care of the authority.

In later years Kahan became an ardent supporter of child-centred residential care and pioneered distance learning for an often ignored and undertrained residential staff. As an advocate of residential care she later wrote one of the seminal investigations of child care in the late twentieth century: the report on the 'Pindown' regime in Staffordshire and the abuses of children in residential care.

A county councillor once said, 'The trouble with Barbara is that she is always on the side of the children.'

Source: Adapted from Philpot 2000.

The young offender

The debate over youth offending is ever recurring, involving questions of causation, analysis of adolescent behaviour, and the most appropriate responses. In Chapter 6 we noted the development of the social conception of delinquency in the years before the Second World War and its genesis in the thinking of William Clarke Hall and Cyril Burt. The preventive sections of the Children and Young Persons Act 1963 reflected an extention of this perspective. By the mid-1960s a 'welfare model' of responses to youth offending had emerged. Offending was regarded as a symptom of deeper maladjustment and family difficulties, and local authority intervention was seen as a therapeutic corrective. The Children and Young Persons Act 1969 as passed by Parliament proved to be the high water mark of the welfare model, committed to providing various forms of treatment rather than punishment for all children in trouble, whether neglected, abused or delinquent. The Act:

- raised the criminal age of responsibility from 10 to 14;
- introduced new grounds for care and supervision orders that applied to young offenders as well as children beyond parental control: exposure to moral danger, found guilty of an offence, beyond parental control or not receiving full-time education;
- provided for 'intermediate treatment' – a group experiences often involving the outdoors or activities that were new to the young person and did not require the making a care order.

The intention was that care proceedings would replace criminal pros-ecution of young offenders and 'treatment' options available to the court. The multiple grounds for care orders however presented a number of diffi-culties that only became more glaring as the 1970s rolled on. The ground of moral danger in practice was applied mostly to girls under 15 deemed 'promiscuous' – boys were rarely so described (Taylor et al. 1979). And in-creasingly the 'offence' condition – some 10,000 young offenders were in care at the end of the 1970s under this provision – was overutilized, relat-ing less to the actual need of the child for 'care and control' than to the magistrates feeling that a care order (and placement in a community home with education) was an appropriate 'sentence' for miscreants even on a young person's first appearance (ibid.: 22). This was the drawback of the welfare model: being placed in care for lengthy periods – often in large, voluntary Victorian 'CHEs' (community homes with education) – having committed only a minor offence. Since they were there ostensibly for 'treatment', the young people tended to languish, waiting for their 18th birthday when the care orders were terminated in any case – a far longer time 'away' than had they gone to a detention centre.

The Act also conferred the right of appeal only on the child; in care proceedings, should the court *not* grant the order, the decision to appeal was left to the child, pitting him or her against their parents. Although formally only the child who had not been made subject of a care order could appeal, the local authority often stepped in to organize that appeal in the child's name, reflecting the reality that care proceedings revolving around neglect were actually between local authority and the parents.

Social workers and probation officers had responsibility for completing social enquiry reports. These were usually drawn up in two major segments: a review of family circumstances and recommendation to the court. The first drew loosely on personality development as shaped by psychodynamic think-ing and often cited problems in the child's background; the second set out the local authority's case for a care or supervision order. There was, as Taylor et al. (1979) pointed out, frequently a collusive relationship between the writer of the report and the magistrates around the decision making. While magistrates were not supposed to know the content of social enquiry reports, research at the time indicated that discussions between the bench and social worker or probation officer often took place.

The broad nature of the grounds for a care or supervision order and the presumption that care by the local authority equated to a kind of therapy, encouraged social workers to confuse the best interests of the child. There was a tendency to conflate the definition of 'best interest' with their own decision regarding what they thought best for a specific child. The notion of applying the 'least detrimental available alternative' formulated by Goldstein et al. (1973) in the United States was generally ignored in the UK. Significantly, that principle would have compelled social workers to ask 'what is it exactly that a care order will provide that the child or young person does not currently have?'

Governmental responses to youth offending continued to vacillate through the 1990s and 2000s between welfare oriented approaches and approaches emphasizing punishment. The murder of two year old James Bulger in 1993 by two ten year old boys, the rise in anti-social behaviour and notions of the 'persistent youth offender' in the mid 1990s brought a 're-penalization' of youth offending. In particular the Crime and Disorder Act 1998 removed the presumption from common law that a child between the age of ten and fourteen was incapable of committing a crime unless specifically proven otherwise (*doli incapax*) and separated the offending child from proceedings that could simultaneously examine his or her welfare.

Yet closer observation of practice on the ground has suggested that members of the multi-disciplinary youth offending teams created by that act, bringing social workers, probation officers and police together, have followed a more open-ended practice that blends punitive and restorative justice perspectives in ways that accommodate elements of the welfare perspective (Burnett and Appleton 2004).

Scotland goes its own way

Scotland avoided many of the above difficulties by creating a new kind of institution: children's hearings for children in trouble. In the wake of interest in preventing juvenile crime in England the Scottish Office (before devolution the principal governmental department overseeing Scottish affairs) established a committee of its own chaired by Lord Kilbrandon to look into the treatment of young offenders and young people in need of care and control. The Kilbrandon Committee – sitting between 1960 and 1964 – picked up the issue that earlier enquiries in England had left to one side: how to devise a system that would deal fairly with both young offenders and neglected young people.

While the Ingleby Committee in England and Wales had focused on the remit of the juvenile court, Kilbrandon's recommendations focused on the *outcome* it wanted for young people and then devised the institution to deliver it. The Committee disposed of the age of criminal responsibility as a 'largely meaningless term' and stated that 'the crime–responsibility–punishment concept may inhibit the court in ordering the treatment the offender needs' (Kilbrandon Committee 1964: para. 54). Whether delinquent or beyond control or neglected, all children in trouble needed 'special measures of education and training, the normal up-bringing process, for whatever reason, having fallen short' (ibid.: 15).

The Kilbrandon Report also rejected the notion of fining parents for their child's misdemeanors. Instead it proposed that *all* children in trouble – whether offenders or in need of care – should, if under 16, be taken out of the court system and transferred to a system of juvenile panels. (The only exception would be those children involved in a serious crime such as murder.) Referral to the panels would only be through the new official called 'the reporter', while the police, local authority and the Royal Scottish Society for the Prevention of Cruelty to Children had their power to initiate proceedings abolished. The reporter became responsible for assessing evidence and deciding whether to proceed to hearing.

The Kilbrandon Committee did not stop there. It also proposed a revamping of social services to fit in with the new approach. Initially it sought to place this new agency within local authorities' education departments because it would be better resourced there. The Social Work (Scotland) Act 1968, however, created a self-standing department with wide responsibilities for child care, child protection, family support and support for older people and adults with disability. Like children's departments in England and Wales the department was empowered to provide assistance to families, either material or in cash, with the latter limited to exceptional circumstances to forestall the local authority greater expense in the future (Murphy 1992).

The panels came into being in 1971 and their influence on youth justice in particular has been profound. In essence the system separated examination of the child's needs from determining guilt. The informal consideration of issues, the involvement of parents and family members, the inclusion of members of the public on the panels were all pathbreaking elements, foreshadowing the idea of family group conferences. Interestingly the grounds for bringing a child before the court are similar to the grounds of the Children and Young Persons Act 1969. Now embodied in the Children (Scotland) Act 1995 they still include the child at risk of moral danger and the child who has committed an offence or is beyond the control of parents.

There were criticisms of the panel system, with a major concern for children who may have been abused by their parents and also on the issue of children's rights where panels have reached decisions regarding a child that the child opposed and which could have gone before a court but did not. Since 1985 the panels have been able to appoint a safeguarder to represent the child's interest. But the percentage of such appointments is small and the issue of whether a panel of untrained persons is able to adequately decide the most complex cases is pertinent.

Child abuse and child protection in the 1970s and 1980s

Child abuse was not a major focus of work for the children's departments set up in 1948 despite the then recent O'Neill case (see earlier this chapter). That changed in the 1960s when Henry Kempe, a paediatrician in Denver looking over radiological evidence, noted numerous fractures old and new in children. Child abuse, he reported, was far more common than thought and was to be found in all social classes. He regarded it as psychological in origin and described a psychotherapeutic treatment regime for abusing parents.

Kempe's findings gained an immediate reception in Britain, particularly from the NSPCC which saw Kempe's work as a way of fending off increasing competition from local authority children's departments by defining a more specialist role for itself (Parton 1979). The NSPCC, following Kempe's suggestion, provided psychotherapeutic counselling and group work for abusive parents, going so far as to establish whole-family residential units. These offered services to only a small fraction of abusive parents. The main impact of Kempe's findings would lay with local authority social work, which by the early 1970s was organized within a social services department. At that point emphasis was on mixed caseloads presenting a wide range of client groups and problems and the acquisition of general or unitary methods. Child abuse had virtually no profile within these developments.

Death of Maria Colwell

The death of Maria Colwell in 1973 very swiftly changed that. Maria died at the hands of her stepfather in Brighton while under local authority supervision. The event initiated a period of media recrimination of East Sussex social services the like of which social work had never encountered before. Led by the Brighton *Evening Argus* but picked up nationally, the stories focused on the shortcomings of the local authority charged with her care. It was a pattern of vilification and accusation that, with variations, was to appear again and again with each succeeding instance of the death of a child under social work supervision. The inquiry into her death noted the lack of communication and inadequate training of social workers with children at risk (Fisher 1974). Olive Stevenson submitted an addendum to the report that remains to this day a celebrated defence of the complexities of social work. She did, however, agree with the enquiry's overall conclusions as to what should be done in the future to avoid such a tragedy.

In terms of professional response, the Department of Health and Social Security (as it was then) made up for lost time by issuing circulars from 1974 onwards which focused on identifying abuse, communication among professionals and management of the response. That response was twofold: getting communication and coordination right among relevant agencies and training key personnel, chiefly GPs and social workers, in the signs and symptoms of abuse. 'Non-accidental injury', a peculiarly negative formulation that nevertheless captured the indeterminate nature of the injury when social

workers and medical practitioners could not be sure whether they were looking at an injury sustained accidentally – falling down stairs for example, being
hit by an older brother, hitting their head while tussling with a friend – or
as the consequence of an assault on a small child. Area review committees
(ARCs) drawn from senior management of health and social services were to
set policy and oversee implementation of that policy. (ARCs were renamed
Area Child Protection Committees in 1988.) Child abuse registers were established containing the names of children which a multi-agency case conference
had concluded had suffered abuse or were at serious risk of abuse.

The most difficult years

Despite the new framework there was a cluster of child deaths in the mid-
1980s – Jasmine Beckford (1984), Tyra Henry (1984), Heidi Koseda (1984),
Kimberly Carlisle (1986), Karl McGoldrick (1986), Liam Johnson (1987),
Sukina (1988) – that set the emotions of the public, media and members of
Parliament on a hair trigger. The vulnerability of the children, the catalogue
of torture and injury, and the lapses of social workers were brought to light in
a series of graphic, detailed enquiries.

These were social work's most difficult years in its entire history. The
excoriation of social work took place within the full glare of national media
which was always prone to work both ends of the decision that faced all social
workers in the field of child protection: criticizing them either for removing
children from fundamentally decent parents or leaving them too long with
monsters. This narrative essentially demanded two contrary perfections in
social work performance simultaneously.

For individual social workers the costs of misjudgement became potential
career wreckers. Guidelines on procedures appeared clear but the complexity
of individual cases outstripped any flowchart, bypassing difficult ethical questions altogether. A large proportion of referral incidents came from parents
themselves (taking their child to casualty) or from neighbours or a nursery.
Checking the central register or invoking a case conference would have the
effect of triggering a formal process, taking away control of the work with the
family from the fieldworker; also fieldworkers at the time felt they had too
little discretion whether or not to call a case conference (Corby 1987). Tough
questions were left for those making the home visit. How far to confront parents with suspicions? How far to be open and above board with the formal
process already under way? How would the social worker maintain a working
relationship despite being the agent of an investigative process over which
parents themselves had little influence and which might end in the removal
of their child? Should there be a sliding scale of official response according to
the severity of the injury?

Lack of written information did not help, whether on the investigatory process itself or explaining to parents that allegations of abuse were just that and that the investigation would be fair and balanced. If suspicions were confirmed, would that mean immediate removal of the child to a safe place as Kempe had urged? If so, should parents be allowed contact (or 'access' as it was called in the 1970s and 1980s) with their child?

Crisis in Cleveland

The crisis in Cleveland was perhaps the single most traumatic event for social work in the second half of the twentieth century. In a few short months – between February and July 1987 – 125 children were diagnosed as sexually abused, with 121 of them by two paediatricians (Butler-Sloss 1988). The children in question came from their own homes, hospital wards, special schools and foster homes. Seventy per cent of the children were immediately separated from their parents by the emergency protection order of the day – the place of safety order which allowed social workers to remove children from their parents' care for up to 28 days. Some of the children were subsequently made wards of court which, prior to the Children Act 1989, was the only means by which the court could attach specific conditions to the child's subsequent care; others were made subject to interim care and supervision orders.

Several elements to this crisis stood out:

- The pediatricians' reliance on a particular diagnostic tool – anal dilatation – which they regarded as a clear indication of penetrative abuse.
- The anger of accused parents who were at times kept in the dark as to what was happening to their children.
- The escalating numbers of children taken into care severely tested local care resources. Professional relationships frayed – for example between police surgeons and the two paediatricians. At the same time pressure built up on the major services as hospital wards filled and social workers rushed to initiate legal procedures. Urgent reactive moves predominated while opinion swiftly polarized between those who thought a kind of hysteria was under way (including the local MP) and those who thought at last the enormity and prevalence of (male perpetrated) sexual abuse of children had been unmasked.[1]

In the end, most of the children involved were returned to their parents as courts began to dispose of the cases. But the crisis affected virtually every dimension of social work with children and families: legal procedures and powers to remove, how far social workers should keep families informed, the reliance on medical diagnosis, the relationships with other professionals.

Lord Justice Butler-Sloss, a leading member of the Family Division, headed the official enquiry into what happened. Her report profoundly affected the way children were subsequently treated during any investigation of sexual abuse allegations. The needs of the children involved had been lost sight of, the report said, and recommended:

- Children are entitled to proper explanation appropriate to their age as to what is going to happen to them, especially if they are to be removed from their home.
- Professionals should listen closely to what the child has to say and the views and wishes of the child be taken into consideration, especially regarding what should happen to the child. These views and wishes should be placed before any court.
- Children should not be subjected to repeated medical examinations for evidential purposes, and, where appropriate, the consent of the child to any examination should be given.
- Children should not be subjected to repeated interviews or interviews of a probing, 'disclosure' kind in which abuse is assumed to have happened. The consent of the child should be gained before interviews are recorded or videotaped.
- Professionals involved should at all times act in the best interests of the child.

Other recommendations suggested that any emergency removal should be for the shortest time possible and access (contact) agreed with parents in writing and only denied in exceptional circumstances. Parents should be informed clearly about what is happening to their child, in writing, and be given support rather than left isolated and bewildered. The trauma of Cleveland revealed how far natural justice principles had been breached in the process of investigation of child sexual abuse.

Key statement from Butler-Sloss

'There is a danger that in looking to the welfare of the children believed to be the victims of sexual abuse the children themselves may be overlooked. The child is a person and not an object of concern.'

Source: Butler-Sloss 1988: 245.

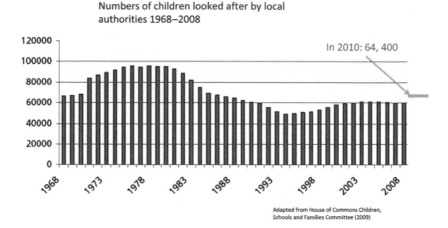

Numbers of children looked after by local authorities 1968–2008

Adapted from House of Commons Children, Schools and Families Committee (2009)

Figure 10.1 Numbers of children in care

Discussion point   Social workers reacting to pressures on child abuse
Look at Figure 10.1. Can you see any rough association between rises in the number of looked after children with major events surrounding child abuse?

Local authority as corporate parent

As the 1970s and 1980s wore on it became more apparent that the 'care' of the local authority often fell well short of helping the child to flourish. Acting as a consistent advocate for the child – ensuring progress in education, creating and sustaining emotional bonds, maintaining links with natural parents, managing relationships with peers, navigating the child through adolescence – all proved difficult.

Research did much to highlight the difficulties around decision making and placement finding. Rowe and Lambert's *Children Who Wait* (1973) called attention to the length of time children in care wait for placement with foster families. Millham and Bullock in their *Lost in Care* (1986) highlighted the number of moves that individual children in care have to make as they shuttle between foster parents and residential establishment (see below). Jackson (1998) called attention to the lack of educational attainment while in local authority care. Evidence also began to accumulate on what happened after a young person left care. Stein (1997) compared what happens to a young person leaving care at age 18 and an 18-year-old leaving home for the first time, with the former shown to be at high risk of homelessness, and social exclusion.

'Permanency planning' was one attempt to create conditions of security and attachments for the child in care. In some local authorities the policy set a six months time limit within which the child would be successfully reunited with their family or have been found a substitute family through long-term fostering or adoption. (In hindsight, six months is not nearly long enough to prepare for and oversee a child's return home, particularly if issues of parental capacity – addiction, learning disability, domestic violence – are involved.)

Moreover, the legal framework based on the Children and Young Persons Act 1969 and the Child Care Act 1980 heavily favoured the local authority at the expense of the parents. It was, for example, entirely within the power of the local authority to deny parental 'access' to their children in their care *without* the matter going before the courts. Other means of contact were either not enabled or were simply refused: exchange of photos, talks with foster parents, opening mail to children in care, supervised access in office, or working with parents to reach satisfactory standards of care and home life in order to have their children back. A child's behaviour during parental visits was often seen as indicative of a problemmatic relationship with parents (Family Rights Group 1986).

Discussion point   Liam

> Liam, nearly FOUR is an intelligent and attractive child with brown eyes, fair skin and light brown hair. His background was English and he lived with his mother who was unable to care for him. Liam is now on a care order and his mother's visits to him are decreasing. We are looking for a permanent home for this small boy which will allow him to be the youngest or only child for some time and enable him to realize his full potential. (Family Rights Group, *Promoting Links: Keeping Children and Families in Touch*, p. 90)

If you were interested in fostering Liam what inferences would you draw from the above short advertisement placed in the local newspaper? Would you assume that Liam's mother was in agreement with the decision to place him long term?

Institutional abuse

In parallel with the deaths of children for whom social services had responsibility a number of incidents of outright cruelty and sexual abuse occurred in children's homes that contributed to a further weakening of public confidence in social work. Frank Beck engaged in brutal assaults on children in the three children's homes he ran in Leicestershire. That he was able to cover his abuse for a time with something he called 'regression therapy' only pointed to the gullibility of senior managers.[2]

Two decades of sexual abuse in children's homes in north Wales finally came to light and gave rise to a public enquiry. The Waterhouse Report on the scandal estimated that some 650 children had been sexually abused over time and recommended that all children's homes have a qualified social worker at their head and that all children have a field social worker who visits them regularly (Waterhouse 2000). (It had often been the case that once a child was in a residential unit field social workers tended to consider that environment safe and the child therefore not requiring regular visits. While not good practice it nevertheless happened widely.)

The scandal in north Wales was only part of the problem. In region after region constabularies were investigating dozens of allegations – in Devon, Manchester, Liverpool, Northern Ireland and elsewhere. This was institutional abuse on a mass scale – all the more shocking because it took so long for senior managers and police to believe that the offending could be so widespread. Children had found it impossible to get a hearing or could not find trusted senior figures who believed what they were saying.

Pindown

The 'Pindown' regime in north Staffordshire homes was another variant of abuse that shook social work to the core. It began as a programme of sanctions in the early 1980s for children who were unruly or had absconded, with consequent 'loss of privileges' but then developed into a regime of harsher treatment. Out of this disciplinary culture a 'special unit' was set up and a 'measures of control' book created to record details of the loss of privileges. As part of the regime children were forced to wear pyjamas during the day and carry out chores.

The phrase 'pindown' was first used – informally without a capital P – in early 1984 – as children new to the home were admitted straight away to the Pindown unit. Three things stand out from the pindown experience. First, that its disciplinary culture fed on itself, becoming more abusive while at times presenting itself as a programme of behaviour modification. This happened as staff appeared to regard the regime as legitimate use of their powers. Second, Pindown's essence was to inflict humiliation on the children, while the children had no one to turn to in confidence, no one to whom they could reveal what was happening. Third, the regime was able to convince senior management of the authority – in so far as it was interested at all – that the regime was making a positive contribution to children's lives. It took some six years for senior management to act, finally picking up on hints and rumours as to what was happening.

An enquiry was finally mounted by Staffordshire Social Services Department in 1990 which investigated the regime, going back to its origins in 1983.

Pindown regime in Stoke-on-Trent children's homes

In the early days of Pindown, before it was called that

> P. [a child] recalled that they were taken to a 'concrete square' and he (Rodriguez) [a member of staff] had us bunny hopping round there. . . . And he had a stick and he was standing there in the middle . . . we had nothing on, just our underpants still, nothing on our feet, and we were bunny hopping round and he was saying move over and he was whipping us, he is mad, but I was laughing, so I was getting it and he was taking it worse because I was laughing. . . . Fundwell [one of the homes] have got up at the top some sheds, garages, actually on the ground. Fundwell workers were actually working there . . . they were up at the top watching it happen they thought it was hilarious.
>
> (Levy and Kahan 1991: 27).

As Pindown became a routine the Levy Kahan report states:

> The log book for 5 March 1984 records that P. a school boy had spent the day before, Sunday, at Duke's Lodge working and that his clothes were wet and dirty but there was no washing powder available to deal with them. The next day there were no toilet rolls available. P. was recorded [by a residential worker] as 'throwing up. I told him to have nothing to eat for 24 hours gave him some milk of magnesia'. There was no suggestion of seeking medical advice.
>
> (ibid.: para. 5.30)

Discussion point   What were they thinking?

Read the above paragraphs about the Pindown regime. Write a short phrase after each that for you sums up the attitude of the residential worker involved.

The Children Act 1989

By the end of the 1980s a number of problems had surfaced simultaneously regarding local authority care and the law on which it was based. These were:

- Parents of children said to be neglected or abused were at a disadvantage compared with the powers of the local authority; these included the 28 day place of safety order, the local council's power to assume parental rights and the multiple grounds on which the local authority could secure a care order.
- Children's own views of what should happen to them in social work decisions were not represented.
- There was no obligation on the local authority to provide family support or to keep parents informed about what was happening to their child in care.
- There was a lack of coordination between private, family law and public law relating to the powers of the local authority and courts.

Calls for major reform of public child care law had been building for some years to deal with these problems before the events in Cleveland, not least from the parliamentary select committee on children in 1984. Then, during what has come to be seen as a period of enlightened national deliberation on children's welfare at the end of the 1980s comparable to that after the Second World War, these issues were addressed in a single package: what was to become the Children Act 1989, which remains, and is likely to remain, the focal point of child law for many years to come.

The Act succeeded in striking a new balance between the claims of family autonomy and those of child protection. It promoted the view that children were best looked after within the family with both parents playing their full part. For the first time the Act provided a checklist in law of what the courts would look to in defining the child's welfare. Crucially it abolished the several grounds for a care order in the Children and Young Persons Act 1969 and replaced them with a single threshold: that the child had or would be likely to suffer significant harm. In addition the local authority would have to convince the court that a care or supervision order for the *specific child* would actually produce improvements in the child's welfare that would otherwise not be obtained if the order were not made. The Act also replaced the place of safety order with the emergency protection order lasting for no more than 72 hours.

In the wake of the Children Act specialization within children's services accelerated.[3] Separate teams were established to undertake family support work as specified in the Act, capable of offering intensive effort to keep children out of care but perhaps with only a single qualified social worker on the team. If a child was to come into care, work with that child would pass to a placement team to oversee a long-term foster placement or adoption. Of course, children themselves did not view the world in terms of such team remits – if the child voted with their feet and went home of their own accord or if the placement broke down, responsibility for the child returned to the family support team.

An assessment team would respond to allegations of abuse sufficiently concerning to require a section 47 enquiry under the Children Act. Its responsibility for children was time-limited to 72 hours, within which time it was expected that a decision would be made regarding the authority's response to the allegation, as required by that section of the Children Act. Only rarely would the team continue to provide advice to the family after that point.

But team remits were fluid and there were further changes as services endeavoured to reflect the complexity of children's lives. Before separate children's services departments were established in 2004, generic 'access' teams managed the 'front door' for all would-be users – receiving and dealing with requests for family support and other services. They had some social workers as members but also relied on knowledgeable but unqualified staff to direct users to the appropriate service. The use of para-professionals, that is, non social workers, in roles that had been previously taken by qualified staff, proliferated particularly within family support teams and among the teams taking on new responsibilities for care leavers which drew heavily on former residential staff (with the closure of homes) and on various community support workers.

Every Child Matters

By the turn of the twenty-first century the Department of Health had committed itself to an ecological assessment of children in need (Department of Health 2000a), a significant step that moved beyond earlier assessments based on developmental milestones and quality of attachment. Children and their parents were now regarded as goal directed, wanting to achieve meaning and a sense of well-being that was not simply a matter of linear progression. As Utting et al. (2002: 12) put it, 'children's wellbeing amounts to more than the successful completion of developmental tasks at different ages and states. Children's wellbeing, or their wellness, is determined by the level of family and community wellbeing.'

Another child's death upended the child care landscape again. Victoria Climbié had been sent from the Ivory Coast to live with her great aunt in London. A year and a half later, in 2000, she died, the result of a catalogue of torture and abuse at the hands of her aunt and the aunt's boyfriend. According to the enquiry into her death there were twelve occasions when the authorities, including social services, could have intervened to save her. Following the recommendations of Lord Laming (Laming 2003), government announced that children's services were to be restructured. The Green Paper *Every Child Matters* and the Children Act 2004 which swiftly implemented it required local authorities to:

- produce an annual children's plan;
- appoint a director of children's services and establish a children's services trust separate from adult services;
- create a statutory safeguarding board with the duty to safeguard children (the area child protection committees which the boards replaced were not statutory bodies);
- gear children's services towards five outcomes which embodied universal aspects of well-being that all children, including children in need, should enjoy, such as staying active and healthy, contributing and participating, and achieving goals;
- embrace data sharing and in particular to deploy a government-created database (Contact Point, now abolished by the coalition government) for use within the common assessment framework.

The overall direction of government thinking – ecological and outcome oriented – prompted debate, particularly within social work education where there were those who argued that children were now more, not less, at risk as a result of the Every Child Matters programme. As Munro and Calder put it in 2005: 'The very words of child protection, child abuse and risk have virtually disappeared from the language, within this agenda victims of abuse are in danger of being lost ... they are being merged with all other groups of children in need (Munro and Calder 2005: 439). (Professor Munro was to be given her chance to reshape this policy when she was appointed by the coalition government to examine child protection in 2010.)

While the Every Child Matters agenda was regarded as root and branch reform, on the ground services had already evolved in its direction. The responsibilities of team structures were not fundamentally changed. Early years services had already developed within local authorities' education services with which social services worked closely to develop a common vision as to what vulnerable children required.

There were drawbacks, however. The potential for tension within the new children's departments formed by the merger of the former social services and education departments as the respective value base of teachers, focusing on stimulating whole-class learning environments and social work focusing on needs of specific children, clashed. In Cheshire the newly appointed director of children's services thought that family centres could close and the work given to Sure Start, overlooking the need for a place to conduct supervised contact between parents and their child in care. Links with adult services were also broken, particularly in relation to parents with disability or drug or mental health problems. Boundary problems between authorities, cost shunting and poor inspection reports also shaped a more defensive posture, with managers having to watch their backs. It was, as one senior manager said, 'A time of blame when mistakes could not be tolerated' (Webb, 2011).

Summary

- The evacuation of children during the Second World War profoundly affected public opinion and led to the creation of local authority children's departments.
- During the 1960s the behaviour of the child as offender and in need of care and control was thought to originate in family problems, with local authority care or intermediate treatment seen as a form of therapy.
- Child abuse was a low priority until the death of Maria Colwell in 1973 after which the Department of Health and Social Security issued regular guidelines for dealing with it.
- From the 1980s on the shortcomings of local authority care became more evident, particularly in loss of contact between children and their parents.
- The Children Act 1989 overhauled earlier child care legislation, giving greater weight to the views of children and families and requiring courts to give first consideration at all times to the welfare of the children before them.

Notes

1. Two books epitomized this conflict: Beatrix Campbell *Unofficial Secrets* and Stuart Bell, MP *Salem Comes to the Boro*.
2. Beck abused, assaulted and raped between 100 and 200 children over a thirteen-year period. He was sentenced to five life terms for sexual assault in 1991 and died of a heart attack in prison in 1994.
3. I am grateful to Margot Webb, former children's manager with Cheshire Social Services Department, for much of the material in this section.

Suggested reading

Hendrick, H. (1994). *Child Welfare in England 1872–1989*. London: Routledge.

Heywood, J. (1959). *Children in Care*. London: Routledge.

Holman, B. (2001). *Champions for Children: The Lives of Modern Child Care Pioneers*. Cambridge: Polity Press.

Packman, J. (1975). *The Child's Generation: Child Care Policy from Curtis to Houghton*. Oxford: Basil Blackwell.

11 From Poor Law to Personalization: Social Work with Adults

In the postwar period social work with adults was still dominated by large institutions and unqualified staff with no focus comparable to the new children's departments. This chapter surveys the patchwork of services and how social work practice only gradually broke free of the legacy of the Poor Law as concepts of community care and individualization evolved.

The chapter covers:

- the postwar development of the mental welfare officer;
- the first moves towards 'de-institutionalization' and community care – bringing people out of psychiatric and long-stay hospitals in the 1960s;
- the effect of the Seebohm reforms on adult services;
- evolution of care management following the NHS and Community Care Act 1990;
- the move towards personalization and individual budgets.

Postwar social work with adults

From the outset the legislation setting up the welfare state divided the care of adults between the National Health Service and local authority health and welfare departments. Part III of the National Assistance Act 1948 gave local authorities the responsibility for providing residential accommodation for those 'in need of care and attention which is not otherwise available to them'. It also required them to provide a range of domiciliary services that included home (or district) nursing and home helps. At the same time the National Health Service Act 1946 – which passed into law in 1948 – made local authorities responsible for arrangements for the care or aftercare of those with mental health problems or learning disability. To do this they established health committees to replace mental deficiency committees and appointed former public assistance personnel as mental welfare officers to carry out the work on the ground.

A rough division of labour emerged: the NHS became responsible for acute and continuing care, and some 90,000 older and disabled people viewed as ill or incapacitated were placed in hospitals. Those needing 'care and attention' (around 42,000) remained under local authority care and were placed in residential homes, very often former workhouses. Local authorities were also encouraged to provide meals, recreational workshops and day centres for older and disabled people.

Within a context of limited resources both the NHS and local authorities had incentives to minimize their budgetary responsibilities. The local authority could from the beginning charge for the day, domiciliary and residential services whereas health services were free to the patient.

Mental disorder and the first phase of community care

The Mental Deficiency Acts of 1913 and 1927 still set the terms for services of people with learning disability while the Lunacy Act 1890 and the Mental Treatment Act 1931 governed the law and practice in relation to people with mental disorder. The Board of Control remained as the national body responsible for setting practice guidance and standards.

Duly authorized officers

The role of the duly authorized officer (DAO) operated under the ethos and legal structures of the prewar Mental Deficiency and Mental Treatment Acts. The officers worked both with people with learning disability and those with mental health problems. They too were engaged in attempts at professional recognition as mental welfare officers – the Mental Welfare Officers Society was founded in 1954 – albeit with virtually no recognized qualifying system to point to. To fill the DAO role for which they were now responsible local authorities appointed largely untrained personnel, including former relieving officers who had at least some experience of the job under the Lunacy Act. They also drew on psychiatric nurses (who were medical and custodial in ethos and resistant to community care ideas). Both groups were largely male. Those coming into the DAO role after the war received cursory on-the-job training. As one recalled some thirty years after being taken on: 'I went to Manchester as a trainee MWO [mental welfare officer] . . . the training consisted of being told: "You really do need to get yourself a pair of stout shoes and an umbrella and you get the No. 53 bus from St. Peter's Square". But that was your training' (quoted in Rolph et al. 2003: 350).

Under the NHS Act the DAOs were given formal responsibility for 'pre-care' (before admission to hospital) and aftercare. The ways of the old regime remained intact. Relieving officers (ROs) before the war had been responsible for compulsory admission to psychiatric hospital but also had some aftercare responsibilities under the Mental Deficiency Acts. Now as DAOs they were given responsibility for home visits to review the circumstances of those learning disabled individuals who were living with their families but who had been ascertained as mentally deficient. Their other duties were to arrange aftercare for those leaving mental deficiency hospitals. But their powers were limited and funding for services non-existent. Their job in the late 1940s involved little more than routine monitoring. Looking back, many testified to the frustration they felt over what there was to offer individual families. As with ROs the DAOs also had a general set of responsibilities in relation to older people and the physically disabled. This role carried over after the Mental Health Act 1959 which gave them a new name – mental welfare officer (Rolph et al. 2003).

Duly authorized officers

In their oral history of mental welfare officers in East Anglia, Rolph and colleagues took testimony from those DAOs practising just after the war.

One remembered:

They weren't very happy times. . . . I used to have a motor-cycle to do my visits, I was in digs and the county council was too mean to give me a telephone, so I found myself, many weekends and bank holidays, having to sit in the office case anybody rang in. . . . I was on call all the time, no standby or payments or relief. . . . A very lonely sort of life. . . . I was only 21.

We did very little work with people with learning difficulties in those days. We kept a Register, but we were run off our feet and the mentally handicapped people very sadly were on the back boiler . . . most of my work was emergency psychiatric. . . . We did do some after-care, but looking back it was pretty primitive.

Others recalled the type of work in relation to clients with mental deficiency:

I used to pop in as part of the mental deficiency list, just spoke to Mrs. So and So. 'Is he alright?' He'd hide away or he'd be down in the garden, but he actually got to know me and he'd come to the garden gate to see me off . . . over the year I got to know him. The doctor who had been looking after that village for years just accepted them as they were, they didn't want to be interfered with, nothing was ever done for him, nothing was ever wanted.

When they ['mental defectives'] were on licence you used to visit them fairly regularly, quite often. I mean in those days you used to handle the odd 'moral defective'. A girl who had a baby was ostracized in the village, used to finish up in the Hospital...you know, never ought to have been there and it was very difficult for them to be discharged.

You had nothing to offer. All you had to offer was that you would see them again in three months or six months' time whenever it was. There was nothing. You would go round, ask the parents how they were, hear various things that had happened in the past three months and then write up your record that you had visited.

Source: Oral testimony from Rolph et al. 2003: 345–6.

'Subnormality' and reference to 'subnormals' and 'mentally handicapped' began to replace the language of mental deficiency and 'mental defective'.[1] Often the work of the DAO was routine: 'Visited, no change' was a common entry found in files. Suspicions around the threats to society that subnormality presented remained: the DAO was often advised to nip any prospective romance in the bud.

For persons with mental health problems there was collaboration with the particular psychiatrists, mental officers of health or county welfare officer to provide greater links with the community. In Suffolk the whole family was regarded as needing support, with the hope that a sufferer could remain at home. In this context the DAO/MWO became more expert at resource finding, developing good relations with other local authority departments such as housing and with voluntary organizations. In Lowestoft, for example, they became adept at lobbying – pushing for funding from many different sources, including private firms in the city – but also setting up an extensive home help service administered by them to support families. In Cambridgeshire, officers attended outpatient clinics with patients and set up the first social clubs for the learning disabled, the so called Bluebird Clubs, funded by the council with both paid and voluntary staff running them (Rolph et al. 2003: 348). Thus a few such localities developed aftercare that foreshadowed some elements of community care, but in general such services were rare.

Mental welfare officers were also expected to work with older people and with the physically disabled on top of their specific duties in relation to those with mental health problems or learning disability. They worked with the blind, the deaf, the elderly, the physically handicapped and the mentally ill – as one testified later to Rolph and colleagues (2003: 353).

Psychiatric social workers

Psychiatric social workers (PSWs) were relatively few in number – in 1950 there were no more than four hundred trained PSWs in Britain. Some two-thirds worked in child-guidance clinics and particular psychiatric hospitals such as the Maudsley in London, with the rest working in the prison and Borstal service or with family agencies such as the Family Welfare Association, child care and care committees (Hunnybun 1950: 105). Within its predominantly psychiatric settings the PSW's role was to take social histories from relatives and discuss with them the arrangements for the patient's care. It also involved helping relatives and friends gain some understanding of the nature of the patient's illness and treatment with a view to winning their cooperation. Direct work with patients was more limited, although their training – with a heavy emphasis on psychodynamic casework – would have suggested otherwise. Part of their work was to talk to ('interview') patients about their general welfare and to arrange to contact the patient once discharged (ibid.).

PSWs had informally struck a kind of bargain: in terms of authority, the psychiatrist and psychiatric hospital management held all the power and influence; within this context the PSW was subordinate but they were in a prestigious line of work and on that basis and on the basis of lengthy specialized training saw themselves as an elite within social work. Obtaining the PSW qualification was difficult and so the number of practitioners was restricted and steeped in psychoanalysis and medical categories.

Social work and reform

By the middle of the 1950s the need for thoroughgoing reform of law, of institutions and of practice in relation to those with mental disorder had become obvious. Several trends contributed to this pressure and were cited in various bills placed before Parliament as the case for reform grew: overcrowding in mental hospitals, shortages of staff, deteriorating buildings that dated from the nineteenth century. The pharmacological revolution was also a powerful trigger for reform, both inside and outside the asylum. Specific drugs – Largactil (Chlorpromazine) was well publicized – controlled mood and diminished aggressive outbursts on the wards, allowing some patients to go home sooner than previously or to remain outside the institution altogether. Very swiftly such drugs came to be regarded as an improvement over the earlier round of invasive treatments such as lobotomy and leucotomy, electroconvulsive therapy and insulin coma therapy. In this context the first real attempt at community care was launched in the late 1950s. Up to that point community-based resources from local authorities were patchy at best – some ran social clubs and offered aftercare support, but local authorities as a whole were new to mental health work. Few employed psychiatric social workers or had sufficient funding to build hostels for short-stay or day centres.

A Royal Commission on Mental Health, convened in the mid-1950s, looked at the sources of stigma associated with mental illness as well as the consequences of the older legislation still in place. Among other recommendations, it called for the abolition of the Board of Control and for local authorities to be given responsibility for organizing preventive services and community care. The Conservative government at the time enacted many of the recommendations in the Mental Health Act 1959. The Act abolished virtually all previous legislation to do with mental deficiency and mental illness. It:

- adopted the term 'mental disorder' to include mental illness, psychopathic disorder and any other disorder of disability of the mind;
- provided the basis for local authorities to establish community care and preventive services such as residential alternatives to hospitals, halfway houses, occupation centres and to appoint mental welfare officers to work in the community;
- established regional mental health tribunals;
- aimed to curtail long periods of hospitalization through reforming the basis for compulsory admission.

Now underpinned by statute, community care was from the first a policy in search of resources. Cost containment was a prime factor, as it would prove to be again in the 1980s. Across the country local authorities received differing amounts of funding to support their new responsibilities which only compounded the highly uneven services already in existence. As a result the bare minimum of resources on which to base community care, such as junior and adult training centres (then often called 'occupation centres') or short-stay hostels, were missing in many areas. In1964 there were still only 31 hostels for those with mental health problems; waiting lists increased and only a 'considerable expansion' would meet the needs of the mentally disordered. Overall local authority expenditure on community mental health remained modest (Welshman 1999). Uneven implementation of community care carried into the 1970s, when non-medical, non-hospital facilities were still deemed rare in a White Paper of 1975. Hospital expenditure continued to dwarf local authority funding of community care. Twenty years after it was announced as official policy, community care was not in any sense a real, funded set of options.

Social workers themselves remained in short supply and, as a key agent of community care, represented an important constraint on development of practice. In 1960, local authorities employed only 26 full-time psychiatric social workers, while a White Paper of 1963 noted that there were only 1,128 social workers in local authorities working in mental health. In 1970 there were still altogether 1,800 social workers in mental health: of these 1,443 were MWOs (and of those only 365 were qualified with the Certificate of Social Work), and 197 were psychiatric social workers (Younghusband 1978).

Mental welfare officers, as the Act now called duly authorized officers, gravitated slowly towards social work training, largely in casework, in the 1960s. Training demanded a sacrifice that only a few officers at the time were able to make for it required moving into lodgings near their training courses, and giving up their local authority salary. In general they were compelled to work on the basis of their own knowledge and experience, including dealing with emergencies. Clarke's account of MWOs working in emergency situations in the late 1960s showed that the number of compulsory admissions was independent of the MWO's level of experience and whether the officer had had specialist training (Clarke 1971).

Mental welfare officers in the 1960s offered essentially a service arranging compulsory admission to hospital, with little in the way of prevention or aftercare. Officers were predominantly male and 'saw their job as controlling and catching "mad" people'; they did not see the task as curative, rehabilitative or therapeutic. As one MWO said: 'it was very rare in those days for people to walk from the house to the ambulance.... [I]t was all arms and legs and being carried.... Then you'd whizz through the streets with ambulance blue lights going. They [the MWOs] were an unstoppable force' (Rolph et al. 2003: 355).

Secondment of personnel from the Mental Welfare Association to local authority health departments brought women into the largely male occupation. Slowly, MWOs began to advocate for patients and move beyond the role of 'handmaiden of psychiatrists' or rubber-stamping GPs' requests for admission. In the 1960s they approached the crisis situation with reluctance and apprehension (Clarke 1971), reducing the decision component to whether or not to admit the patient. Their growing ambivalence towards hospitalization was reinforced by the anti-psychiatry movement (see below), which was strongly suspicious of the power of institutions.

Anti-psychiatry movement

The strongly libertarian, individualist element in the anti-psychiatry movement was explicit in the work of Thomas Szasz, whose *The Myth of Mental Illness* (1960) and later publications also made an impact. Szasz offered strong criticism of medical practice and its tendency to identify as illnesses behaviour that arose from what he called 'the problems of living'. He was strongly critical also of psychiatry's powers to involuntarily incarcerate people in mental hospital and to undertake other forms of 'treatment' of psychosis such as electroconvulsive therapy and lobotomies. Szasz was one of the first to offer a comprehensive critique of the 'medical model' and the way it approached social problems and social behaviour – all the more notable because he launched it at a point when medicine was unchallenged in its authority and public regard. He was also one of the first to note the power of words and how important the contest over rival sets of vocabularies is – for example, who gets to apply the word 'sick' to specific forms of behaviour. In this he anticipated, at least in the anglophone world because it had not yet been translated, the work of his contemporary, Michel Foucault, who addressed some of these same themes.

Even more influential was Erving Goffman's analysis of the 'total institution' (1961). He wrote:

> [T]otal institutions disrupt or defile precisely those actions that in civil society have the role of attesting to the actor and those in his presence that he has some command over his world – that he is a person with 'adult' self-determination, autonomy and freedom of action. A failure to retain this kind of adult executive competency, or at least the symbols of it, can produce in the inmate the terror of feeling radically demoted in the age-grading system.
>
> In general, then, mental hospitals systematically provide for circulation about each patient the kind of information that the patient is likely to try to hide. And in various degrees of detail this information is used daily to puncture his claims. At the admission and diagnostic conferences, he will be asked questions to which he must give wrong answers in order to maintain his self-respect.
>
> (Goffman 1961: 148–9)

While few MWOs embraced fully the tenets of anti-psychiatry, a broader range of criticism and consensus was emerging as to how those with mental health problems should be treated. There was concern with individual civil rights of those compulsorily admitted to hospital, especially their loss of freedom, on the one hand and the risks posed to the community at large, on the other. Long-stay hostels along the lines of therapeutic communities run by the Richmond Fellowship, MIND and other voluntary agencies carved out a highly supportive environment that was nevertheless neighbourhood based.

By the 1980s it was clear that community care for those with mental health problems was falling far short of its objectives. Between 1978 and 1991 the number of psychiatric beds had fallen from 89,000 to 50,000, a decline of some 44 per cent, yet community-based resources remained relatively sparse. While some sixty hospitals had closed altogether there was no evidence that the funding was redirected to building up community services. By 1991 only nine pence out of every pound spent on care for those with mental ill-health went to local authorities; the rest went to national health (Eaton 1994). The right of sufferers to any kind of local provision rested on old legislation: for accommodation on Part III of the National Assistance Act 1948 which obliged local authorities to provide residential accommodation for those who 'by reason of age, illness, disability or any other circumstances are in need of care'; and for day activities or help inside the home, on the Chronically Sick and Disabled Act 1970 which obliged authorities to provide 'services' for those who are 'blind, deaf or dumb or who suffer from mental disorder of any description'. Neither pathway was productive; rates of homelessness among those discharged from psychiatric hospital soared.

Forceful campaigns for improvement in community care came from across the voluntary sector and advocacy groups. MIND was perhaps the most prominent but by no means the only organization in promoting community-based initiatives for survivors. MIND, for example, campaigned for:

- 24-hour access to services for those in crisis;
- wider availability of counselling and other talking treatments;
- national standards for community care services;
- an end to dangerous prescription of psychiatric drugs;
- reduction in the use of electroconvulsive therapy and its total ban for children (Sayce 1994).

By the end of the 1980s, as the era of key workers and case managers was dawning, those examining the role of social work in the field began to think that what was needed was an independent advocate rather than a practitioner limited by role in a hospital or social services department. The question remained whether that would happen given the fact that mental health legislation had consistently assigned functions in relation to compulsory admission to social workers and their predecessors.

Older people and the second phase of community care

By the mid-1980s of 3 million people aged over 75 – some 300,000, or 10 per cent of the age group were in homes or long-stay beds in hospitals. In the face of an underfunded community care infrastructure and pressure to reduce long-stay patients in hospitals, government began to finance the care of older people through social security between 1983 and 1993 in private residential homes. These homes soon became the main provider of convalescence, rehabilitation and long-term nursing and residential care. Expenditure rose exponentially, from £39 million in 1982 to £253 million in 1992. The full costs of private nursing or residential care could be claimed by an individual solely on the basis of financial need.

Whether the person actually needed that care was not considered in any formal way. Older people were choosing residential care simply because there were no community-based options (Rummery and Glendinning 1999). Many applicants for residential care, shocked by a traumatic fall or bereavement, had not received the information they needed to make an informed choice (Neill et al. 1986), nor were they given the chance to visit the home beforehand. A survey at the time by the National Institute for Social Work found that a high proportion of applicants for both private and local authority homes applied only reluctantly, were not very disabled and had not received or even been offered intensive services prior to admission (NISW 1988). Anxiety about risk, especially felt by carers and family, as well as stress felt by carers and neighbours who had become exhausted or faced multiple responsibilities, lay behind a high proportion of applications.

Lapses in social work assessment were also part of the broader system which relentlessly pushed older people towards residential accommodation: admissions were made on the basis of emergency, treatable health problems were overlooked, and full, functional, medical and social assessments were comparatively rare. In the assessment process social workers typically would see the applicant only once and the carer not at all. As a result, specific difficulties and wishes of the key parties would not be identified and remediable problems missed (NISW 1988: 13–14).

There were further questions over the standards of residential care itself. To examine the entire sector the Independent Review of Residential Care was commissioned in late 1985 – the Wagner Committee named after its chairperson, Gillian Wagner – which reported some two years later. The report itself made a powerful plea for gearing residential care to the individual. It could do this by giving residents the right to exercise choice over their lifestyle, continuing links with their previous life and creating an ethos based on shared values. The report particularly emphasized that the more personal the issue was the more choice residents should have, for example over relationships, personal space, physical care and food (Wagner 1988: 62).

The Wagner Committee hears from a relative

In taking testimony from around the country the Wagner Committee noted that it was often little things in residential regimes that hurt but would have been relatively easy to fix. A relative wrote to the Committee:

> It has always been rather sad to see him clad in clothes other than his own (which are well-labelled and all co-ordinating). To see him eat, using old, worn second grade cutlery, drink from a plastic cup, all presented on a rather grotty tray, can be so upsetting and served to add salt to a wound for me or his wife when visiting, after spending a life together since the age of seventeen. Having enjoyed all the niceties of life in their home together, these standards are humiliating and degrading.
>
> (Wagner 1988: 61)

Lack of choice, lack of security and absence of any sense of control by individual residents over their lives, these were the chief deficiencies found across private and local authority homes. Within social work there were calls for more comprehensive, multidisciplinary assessments, for greater individuality and for control to pass to users. Mary Marshall stressed the importance of understanding older people's social history and the value of a lifetime's social and familial connections. Moreover, social workers needed the capacity to undertake a careful assessment of needs and risk in one visit to forestall having a chain of various agencies visiting to put together a composite judgement. Above all, social workers should have the capacity to handle crises – preserving time to decide, to inform, to choose and above all to avoid emergency admissions (Marshall 1983).

NHS and Community Care Act and the care management role

The NHS and Community Care Act 1990 (NHS CC Act) and the tasks that followed from it owed much to the concept of case management as it had been elaborated through the previous decade chiefly in the United States where it had arisen within a fragmented provider environment. The overall aim was to maintain the integration of older people in society by promoting independence and strengthening their networks to relieve the burden on carers.

Case management in this first version aimed to stimulate the more efficient use of resources and to improve flexibility and field-level coordination among services drawing on the wide range of resources available (Davies 1992: 2–3). Case management, it was argued, provided a body of logical tools and experience about how to link arrangements, resources and practice:

- case-finding by which the means identifying those who would benefit most from the agency services;
- screening for eligibility;
- assessment, linked to specific purposes;
- care planning and reviewing, and adjustment to those plans as needed (Davies 1992: 8).

The NHS CC Act reshaped case management (renaming it care management), and in doing so changed the function of social workers in England and Wales. Previously, local authority provision dominated services for adults and, with social workers performing roles such as gatekeeping resources and maintaining overview of care, these regimes were still largely underpinned by local authority providers. The actual assessment of need and subsequent provision of service, whether home care, day centre or residential placement, were carried out by social work assistants or home care organizers. Prior to 1990, entry to private residential care seldom involved a social worker. There was a relational component to these roles, with assessors developing relationships with individual families and discussing their needs in an informal casework role.

While the government's objective was to discover the individual needs of users and to not prejudge those needs purely in terms of the residential or day centres run by local authorities, it was also clear that resources and funding for meeting those needs were not unlimited and that local authorities had to strike a balance between their assessment process and the claims on resources that their individual assessment of individuals would entail. The Department of Health issued firm guidance outlining what care management involved. Assessment, it said, is an integral part of care management, but is only one of the seven core tasks. From the outset the Department regarded 'need' as a complex and dynamic concept (and said as much in its guidance to managers and practitioners), varying according to changes in legislation and local policy as well as available resources and patterns of local demand (Department of Health 1991: 10).

In addition, the NHS CC Act charged local authority care managers with expanding the 'independent sector' – the private and voluntary providers of community care services. While that had happened already in terms of private residential establishments for older people, the Act was intended to give support to local voluntary bodies that had supplied day and support services backing up the local authority. Some 85 per cent of the transitional grant coming to authorities as the Act was implemented had to be spent on the independent sector, which included arm's length trusts set up to run former local authority homes, and housing associations that wished to develop care services (Bamford 2001: 13).

From our vantage point today, the NHS CC Act was a watershed that changed utterly the direction of social work with adults.[2] But on the ground it did not at first appear that way. As the date for implementation approached – 1 April 1993 – local authorities were in vastly different positions in their response to the Act. Some organized an operational network of senior managers to examine the financial implications of the Act and to explore the implications of the care manager's role. Others made no preparation at all, and as late as the end of the 1990s were still regarding their own residential and day care facilities as essentially predetermining what a person's 'need' was. While health authorities had a good grasp of the health needs of the population as a whole in their area, few social services departments had equivalent studies available that would provide them with a snapshot of the needs of different adult user groups. The Audit Commission (1986) had urged dividing population projections at least into low and high public sector dependency needs (the first a much larger number than the second), yet little advance work had been done (Webb 2011).

Neither the purchaser–provider split nor the 'internal market' was a prominent consideration in the minds of practitioners in the early years of implementation. Commissioning and expanding the provider market was slow to develop as part of the care manager's role. In arranging care for older people, private residential homes had already come to replace a great many lo-cal authority 'elderly persons homes', and the once public service had already been privatized. Other forces also made the Act feel less like a revolution: discussions with users about charging for services was already part of the con-versation with users, one that social workers were uncomfortable with to the extent that they would downplay the subject (Webb 2011).

There were frank admissions that social work was not ready for the role of care manager – that social work with adults had not developed a body of knowledge on which to base authoritative practice, with the possible exception of mental health. As a result, in practice social workers were not going out to assess needs with a blank piece of paper but were, as in the past, responding to a referral from hospital, GP or relative that the person 'needs day care' or 'needs residential care'. In many authorities, adults in hospital but in need of care still went straight into residential units as they always had done. For health authorities and hospital managers, community care meant little more than 'out of hospital'.

While there was potential to shape the form and values of care manage-ment on the ground, social work was not in a position to capitalize on it. While some authorities focused on 'purchasing' as part of the care manager role, such moves failed to deliver visible improvements in the independent sector. This eventually persuaded authorities to integrate purchasing with a broader role – commissioning. In that role, care managers became involved in partnerships with users to determine levels of need and the best ways to meet those needs. By 2000 this was moving towards greater individual con-trol – pressed especially by disability advocacy groups. The Direct Payments Act 1996 – providing funding directly to users that had previously gone to the local authority to provide care – proved to be only the first step in a process that became more pronounced after the turn of the twenty-first century. Com-missioning also involved roles new to social work: understanding costs and recognizing when costs are unrealistically low or high, and knowledge of the market, that is, the current mix of public, voluntary and private provision, and to know the strength and weaknesses of these providers (Bamford 2001: 15).

꙳ One of the consequences of the NHS CC Act was a move from universal access to NHS services based on comprehensive universal rights to health care, to discretionary access to what had already become underfunded, residual lo-cal authority services. New charging tariffs by local authorities also meant that chronically ill people and those with disability reliant on local authority day and domiciliary care, would be means tested for a service, should they be pro-vided with one. The introduction of market reforms and contracting services produced organizational cultures in which gatekeepers kept close scrutiny on the difficulties of specific individuals to see if the funding responsibility should actually be theirs or not. Organizational boundaries and responsibilities were demarcated more closely, cost shunting more prevalent, and collaborative arrangements, particularly between health and the local authority, more difficult to maintain.

Personalization and social care for adults: the third phase of community care

It took a full decade for practice around community care to mature. Two imperatives, at times conflicting, at times working in tandem, dominated the post-2000 world of social care and profoundly affected the shape and availability of community care in the first decade of the twenty-first century: (i) scarcity of resources, which dictated the need for eligibility criteria, and (ii) personalization and individual control by the citizen user.

Eligibility criteria

Unlimited funding for all levels of social care needs was beyond the reach of any authority, subject as it was to central government spending reviews and grant allocations. Rules for eligibility were crucial to the rationing of services. In the first years of implementation of the NHS CC Act each authority tended to set its own criteria for services. The White Paper *Modernising Social Services* (Department of Health 1998) noted that this variability of criteria and the apparent reluctance to review them produced gross inequalities across the country. The tendency for local authorities to have different criteria for eligibility for assessment and for services was additionally confusing. In response, the Department of Health issued *Fair Access to Care Services* (FACS) in 2003, setting out bands of eligibility criteria common to all authorities. FACS was more than a guide – local authorities were not to vary the wording: once a council had decided what it could afford for social care, it was to use the exact wording of the band to describe the risk factors from which eligible needs would be identified. Although FACS was not expected to bring about similar decisions across the country, it was designed to ensure equal treatment of need. The difference between 'critical' as a category of need – when life was under threat or significant health problems had developed or serious abuse was occurring – and 'substantial' was only one of degree, but often precisely the difference between receiving and not receiving a service.

Personalization

The principle of putting services at the command of the adult who receives them is the other major driving force behind change in social care in the twenty-first century. It draws on theories of citizenship, consumer choice, and autonomy, and in practice aims to give individuals sufficient control of resources to shape the care that they determine they need. One word has captured this complex notion: 'personalization'. In one sense it continues an implicit line of development begun with the NHS CC Act, through direct payments initiatives and the opening up of care services to diversity. It is fully articulated in the ministerial concordat *Putting People First* and in associated guidance from the Department of Health from 2007 on. As Leadbetter (2004: 2) observed, personalization 'only tends to work in services that are face to face, based on long term relationships and which depend on direct engagement between the providers and users'. Personalization does accept that adults are their own best experts and have the most knowledge regarding their needs. From that flows the idea that practitioners have to become advisers, advocates, solutions assemblers and brokers (ibid.).

Within the move to direct control by individuals in making their own care arrangements social work has at times struggled to find a distinctive role for itself as opposed to the other sources of support open to adults – peer groups, family relations, care support groups, and other professionals particularly in health. It has had to re-emphasise that it is a regulated graduate profession with a code of practice and constantly developing knowledge base with a key role in public protection. A recent statement on the social work contribution to personalization, using language that could have been found in any similar statement over the past twenty years, highlighted its capacity to:

- build professional relationships and empower people as individuals in their families and communities;
- work through conflict and support people to manage their own risks;
- support people with assessment of their needs, circumstances and options;
- work with families to improve and safeguard vulnerable family members.

The same publication states that social work also provides 'early intervention and preventive services, and inclusion and helping to build capacity, social enterprise and social cohesion' (ADASS 2010: 3). As so often in the past, aspiration runs high but there are implicit questions over whether these are in any way unique.

Other changes under the banner of personalization have included setting up of call centres and disbanding emergency duty teams – leading in Liverpool, for example, to a bitter three-month strike in 2004 as social workers protested against what they considered a debasing of social work values and service and the fact that the local council was arguing that those staffing the call centre did not have to be qualified.

The historical lack of integration of adult care services, particularly between health and social services, has undermined implementing personalization in the face of scarcity and economic crisis. *Putting People First* envisaged a tightly integrated community-based service in which no adult with social care needs was to be cut adrift. The local authority was designated to be the agent of change to meld third sector (civil society) organizations, private services, NHS services and other statutory agencies into a seamless care network delivering certain outcomes: to allow individuals to live independently, to recover quickly from illness, to exercise maximum control over their life and that of family members, to prevent children taking on inappropriate caring roles (Department of Health 2007: para. 3.2). Common assessment, person-centred planning, self-directed support and personal budgets were the means by which social workers and social care personnel would bring this about.

Deprivation of liberty and safeguarding

The power to detain, to restrict the liberties of an adult citizen, marks the counterpoint to community care – but is closely intertwined with the success or failure of that policy. The more reliant on community-based services for vulnerable adults the more the need for sensitive, accurate responses to those individuals who cannot survive in their community or who become a danger to others. Social workers with adults have long had powers to remove individuals from their homes and families in order to safeguard their health. While used rarely, powers under the National Assistance Act 1948 provided the grounds for taking individuals at risk to places of safety, in particular older people who did not fall under the Mental Health Acts. The more widely used power to detain adults was in the field of mental health, but there has always been overlap in application of both sets of powers now acknowledged in the Mental Capacity Act 2005 which sets out specific grounds and procedures for the deprivation of liberty.

Deprivation of liberty and adult with mental health problems

The number of psychiatric beds in England has fallen from a peak of 150,000 in 1955 to 28,000 by 2007, giving a rough indicator of the extent of community care provision. High-profile instances of violence committed by those under supervision in the community and the incidence of self-harm and suicides, together with high rates of homelessness of those discharged from hospitals, have formed a kind of undertow to the general policy. For social workers this has increased focus on risk management – amid perceptions that different groups are more, or less, suitable to community care. There is, for example, a pronounced gendered dimension to this: women are regarded as more suitable, men as disproportionately 'mad and dangerous' (Payne 1999).

In the 1970s, MIND began to campaign for better protection of patients' rights; its efforts coincided with BASW's call to clarify and professionalize the role of social workers in relation to mental health legislation. As a result the Mental Health Act 1983 created the approved social worker (ASW) as key to the process of removing a person compulsorily to psychiatric hospital, with an inbuilt guarantee of special training for those to be designated as ASWs. Both aspirations had already been presented in MIND's submission to the Department of Health and Social Security by the transplanted American Larry Gostin (Gostin 1975: 36). Writing almost a decade later in *Social Work Today*, Gostin reaffirmed his belief in social workers as advocates: 'While the social work profession is not responsible for laws and social attitudes affecting the liberty and autonomy of their clients, they can take on a central role in defending their clients' rights' (Gostin 1984: 16).

The introduction of the ASW did not have the intended impact on the field of mental health. Patients continued to be in a weak position when it came to obtaining services, whether these were hospital based or community based. Prior (1992) argued that this disappointment arose from the inherent contradictions in the role of the social worker. The discretionary powers on the ASW in England and Wales in the Mental Health Act 1983 (and for Scotland and Northern Ireland in the succeeding years) set up potential conflict with the nearest relative who had long held similar powers under the older legislation. (Interestingly, MIND actually campaigned for the elimination of the role of nearest relative – a move which government firmly rejected.)

The Act also put social workers in conflict with public interest, or rather with the public's perception of that interest which might favour compulsory admission when other forms of at-home care were appropriate. This proved a difficult balance between what was least restrictive care for the patient on the one hand, and protection of the public on the other – with social workers mediating, finessing and brokering that balance.

The creation of the ASW role highlighted some of the pitfalls of upgrading specific roles in social work. To become an ASW was a reasonable aspiration as it would confirm the expertise of practitioners who were already crisis experts and who would not simply rubber-stamp the decisions of others (*Community Care*, 1982). But the new role required additional post-qualifying training in mental health on CCETSW-approved programmes, with the names of success-ful candidates entered onto a central register.

Yet there were difficulties. The local government officers' union NALGO noted that the proposed training and assessment of ASWs would change con-ditions of service for its members and placed a ban on its members taking the CCETSW examination. The union's argument was that social workers 'who had been carrying out similar functions under the Mental Health Act 1959 were now being faced with the prospect of being trained and assessed (with the possibility of failure) for these aspects of their work' (*Community Care*, 1 March 1984, p. 6). To make the new law work, four thousand social workers had to be brought in under transitional arrangements. The episode showed the dilemmas that social work faced in achieving specialist recognition for particular expertise but doing so in a way that was fair to the workforce as a whole.

Summary

- For a decade after the Second World War social work practice was still largely governed by laws, concepts and terminology dating back as much as sixty years before.
- There was no reform in adult social care comparable to that in children's services.
- Community care policies were initially pursued in relation to adults in large psychiatric hospitals – the result of financial pressures, the pharmacological revolution and concern that large institutions were dehumanizing. But the policies were underfunded and local authorities slow to provide community-based facilities to support the programme.
- Social workers involved in mental disorder – duly authorized officers and, after the passage of the Mental Health Act 1959, mental welfare officers – were often unqualified throughout the 1960s.
- A second phase of community care – sparked initially by the inadvertent government funding of private residential care home places through the social security payments in the 1980s – resulted in revolutionary changes to social work with adults following the introduction of care management role in the NHS and Community Care Act 1990.
- A third phase of community care has taken the individualization of the vulnerable adult as consumer to its logical conclusion – with provision of individual user budgets.

Notes

1. The term 'handicap' is said to derive from the Elizabethan practice of licensing particular individuals to collect alms from passers-by in a cap.
2. For this section I am indebted to John Webb, former director of adult services at the Wirral. In our wide-ranging conversation he made many of the points I draw on here.

Suggested reading

Department of Health (1991). *The National Health Service and Community Care Act: Practitioner's Guide*. London: Department of Health.

Gostin, L. (1977). *A Human Condition*. London: MIND.

Leadbetter, C. (2004). *Personalisation*. London: Demos.

Welshman, J. (1999). 'Rhetoric and reality: community care in England and Wales 1948–1974', in P. Bartlett and D. Wright (eds) *Outside the Walls of the Asylum: Community Care 1750–2000*. London: The Athlone Press.

For an insight into psychiatric hospitals in the mid-1950s go to the valuable Pathé news archive at http://www.britishpathe.com/record.php?id=40676. And for an unsparing look at a mental hospital regime around that time – admittedly French but certainly illustrative – go to http://www.britishpathe.com/record.php?id=67591.

12 Conclusion: Understanding Social Work History

The main objective of this volume has been to familiarize readers with the context and content of the development of social work – with the people and practice as it evolved over a century and a half and more. The goal was to get readers thinking for themselves about the overall sweep and significance of social work's history. In doing this I have kept any hints of a broader interpretation of this history to a minimum. This concluding chapter aims to fill that gap, if tentatively, by suggesting ways in which the development of social work can be understood. It seeks to do three things:

- to pull out the major recurring themes from the past that are likely to resurface in the future;
- to discuss and evaluate various single-narrative interpretations of social work history;
- to consider certain issues and conundrums that social work has had to face and will face in the future.

Recurring themes in social work history

The familiar claim that people make history but not always as they would wish is as true for social work as for any other human endeavour. The present is not a blank sheet on which things may be designed from scratch but is constrained by entrenched patterns and ways of thinking – what some social scientists have called 'dependency pathways'. It is important therefore to identify certain recurring themes in the history of social work that are likely to impact the future in one form or another.

Defining social work

Attempts to define social work, whether for the public or its own sense of professional understanding, are a regular occurrence. Many hands have had a stab at it: definitions of casework in the early twentieth century, the Younghusband Report of 1959, BASW's definition of the social work task in the 1970s, the Barclay Report, the competences and skills identified in the 1980s before the DipSW was introduced, the consultant's definition of social work before the degree was introduced in the late 1990s and, more recently, the Social Work Task Force. This tells us one thing: that pinning down what social work does in a concise way is extremely difficult. Each generation – or half-generation – tries to find its own language. The assumption seems to be that there must be a formula in words and that unless social work is defined pithily it is not a significant activity. Each definition in its time has been largely accepted by social workers themselves but has rarely been uncritically accepted by other professionals or the public at large.

This raises the question, what if social work cannot be defined? Perhaps attempts at definition are looking in the wrong place. To a certain extent social work takes on the colour of its context; in any case it is clear that from the beginning social work was an *ensemble of functions* in a way that nursing for example is not. At the very outset social work was defined philosophically by the leading public intellectuals of the Charity Organisation Society (COS) which connected its casework activity to an organic and ethical view of society. But from our vantage point we can see that a number of other organizations were also then engaged in social work. By 1900 moral welfare with unmarried mothers, the Church of England temperance volunteers who became the first probation officers, relieving officers for the local boards of guardians, inspectors for the NSPCC, care committee workers were all clearly carrying out social work functions of contact, protection, relationship building, support and advice – the great proportion as volunteers. No single bottle (or definition) would have been big enough to put that diverse, multifaceted genie of social work back into.

As it matured, social work acquired other functions, functions that it in part sought for itself (with the 'mentally deficient') and in part were given to it, for example care committee organizers suddenly given immense responsibilities for evacuated children during the Second World War, the transference of responsibility for child neglect from the voluntary sector to local authority in the 1930s or care management tasks in the 1990s.

It is true that there are consistent elements that can be extrapolated from the ensemble of specific functions: it combines everyday experience and understanding of human behaviour, with lengthy training in law, procedure, detection and the capacity to work under great stress. But any definition based on these will last only until new tasks and functions cause it to go out of date. Perhaps, then, social work does not lend itself to a single definition; perhaps it is a protean profession – adapting, changing shape, responding in different guises as the need requires with an evolving value base that provides a compass.

For the past two decades social work, that is, the ensemble of functions and roles, has again become dispersed and no longer wholly owned by those with the title of 'social worker'. Currently, family support workers, job advisers working with those on incapacity benefit, refugee agencies supporting asylum seekers, private family placement agencies, supported housing units, voluntary agencies dealing with young people with mental health problems, all have personnel carrying out social work functions.

Quest for professional status

Closely tied to attempts to find a single definition has been the effort to secure professional status. This has been a century-long quest, inching forward here, getting knocked back there and, until 1970 at least largely based on separate organizations representing specialist social activity – almoners, child care officers, moral welfare workers and others.

Being 'professional' is one thing – it calls to mind competent practitioners validated and secure in their approaches, carrying out their job to a high standard. A recognized 'profession' is something quite different. Its traits are acknowledged to be:

- authority derived from the public's trust in its expertise;
- lengthy training to qualify;
- self-regulation by an organization that speaks unequivocally for the practice and the body of practitioners willing to give allegiance to that organization;
- conduct based on an ethical code (Friedson 1970).

Social work has taken steps in relation to all four of these points in the past forty years but is still well short of securing full professional status, particularly in relation to the first and third points above. In the 1950s and the 1960s the prospect seemed within reach – the Association of Child Care Officers came as close as any social work organization to achieving essential public respect. Other professional associations, such as the Institute of Psychiatric Social Workers, saw themselves as an elite but were small in number and, as Abraham Flexner said so many years ago, often acted as adjuncts to more powerful and well established professions (Flexner 1915).

The formation of the British Association of Social Workers (BASW) in 1970 held out further promise but there were difficulties for by this point social work itself was divided over whether it wanted to be a profession or an occupation, a conflict of perspective that continues to this day. There were a number of ingredients to this conflict – BASW faced difficult dilemmas, as discussed in Chapter 8, that caused it to manoeuvre pragmatically (or expediently in the view of some). There was, and continues to be, heartfelt uncertainty as to how far becoming a profession would distance social work from those it works with. In the 1970s, persuasive arguments were made that a profession's power was based on rigorously controlled entry to its ranks, and on its members holding exclusive knowledge that only they can interpret. Do professional aspirations then fit with democratic aspirations? Can a hierarchy of power and influence be squared with commitments to equality and anti-oppression strategies? Is the essence of social work defined by its qualification or by its employment? (Bilton 2011).

The uncertainty surrounding the College of Social Work is only another reminder that, at best, social work is a 'semi-profession' or a 'bureau profession' with some elements of a profession blended within bureaucratic performance. The various Royal Colleges of medicine are places of intellectual rigour, continuing research and fellowship; their members continue to practise throughout their career. Becoming a member *is* induction into the profession – where standards of practice are expected to be high and support always available (Hanvey 2011). While the College of Social Work may offer some of these attributes (of course, they take decades to build up), the question is whether it has the autonomy of a Royal College and whether social workers will regard it with the same commitment and loyalty as, for example, paediatricians regard their Royal College of Paediatrics and Child Health (ibid.).

The market and the public sector

Argument over the rival virtues of public sector social care provision and market-provided social care services is the principal contest of our time and has been under way for at least twenty years. Other issues are subordinate to this. As we have seen, the mechanisms for submitting social care and social work services to market disciplines began in the wake of the NHS and Community Care Act in the early 1990s. The effect of that Act was not a thunderclap but a slow unfolding of a logic that has only gathered pace in the intervening twenty years. As we noted in Chapter 9, social services departments adapted step by step at first. The process accelerated under Labour and again under the coalition government elected in 2010.

Several important questions arise as a result. Where should the boundary between state-provided services and market-provided services lie? Is there an optimum balance in the 'mixed economy of care' or is that simply a euphemism for a continuous process of moving services out of the public sector? Do state-provided services have intrinsic virtues that market-provided services do not have? Conversely, do they have intrinsic defects? And on the other side of the coin, do services provided through market mechanisms have defects or virtues? There are no automatic answers to the above questions but they require further thought, research and deliberation. Once social workers would have looked to the great theorists and proponents for social democracy – Townsend, Titmuss, Marshall – and confidently called for a return to a refreshed public sector. That option is no longer available: market principles are entwined and welfare reform makes work, not citizenship, the basis for any entitlement to benefits.

In provision of care we have moved deeply into market-providing territory. The question is, how far can the market be relied upon to supply quality care? Years ago, economists noted that while many sectors of the economy may improve their productivity, care services cannot do so. They are labour intensive, they rely on face-to-face contact and person-specific knowledge that cannot be standardized or depersonalized. Labour costs – the pay of care workers – cannot easily be cut without drastically reducing either the number of carers or the quality, skills and sensitivity of carers, or both. In such an environment, care becomes a commodity, one moreover often purchased for a person in need by others – commissioners or family members – who find it difficult to monitor the quality of the care since they are not the ones experiencing it.

Social exclusion and social work

Urban poverty arising from rapid industrialization was the midwife of social work: no poverty, no social work. And if there is one unvarying thread in social work history it is that poverty, disadvantage and exclusion dominate the lives of users. Of course, individual habits, morals, weaknesses, impairment and illness have played a large part in those who seek – or who are compelled to accept – social work services, and social work history offers a laboratory on what happens when practitioners focus only on the personal without taking the social, economic and neighbourhood dimensions of the individual's life into account.

Tackling the roots of exclusion by attempting to broaden the scope of social work to include neighbourhood-level intervention of one kind or another is a regular feature of this history. The settlement house movement, the civic culture of the guilds of help in the early twentieth century, preventive work in the 1960s, radical social work's liking for community development in the 1970s, community social work in the 1980s, family support measures for children in need and anti-racist work in the 1990s, all embraced the idea.

Like Sisyphus in the ancient Greek myth, social work has had to push the boulder of community-level interventions to tackle structural sources of disadvantage many times up the long hill only to watch it come rolling down to the bottom again. Opposition always materializes. This reaction is sometimes in the realm of ideas, for example Pinker's influential argument against community social work in the early 1980s. Sometimes it arises from political hostility, whether from Labour councillors who do not relish local community development roles materializing on their patch or from Conservative councillors who want social workers to respond only to those most in need and then only when those persons are individually in deep trouble. Sometimes opposition comes from within social work itself, from those who think that engaging in working with people in larger groups is getting into territory best left to others. But the history suggests that the stone will be pushed up the hill once more by some, if not all.

No conclusive solutions – only pendulums

One of social work's historical functions is to act as navigator, resource manipulator and broker to assist people through the complexities of benefits, community care, child care procedures or a half a dozen other systems that require a pilot. As such, practitioners are forever having to change tack, caught in winds that suddenly change direction, that damn them if they do and damn them if they don't. The pendulum swings back and forth between supposed solutions to intractable problems or between social policy goals. This phenomenon is most apparent on the question of whether to leave children at risk with their families or to remove them. Department of Health policy has pointed one way and then the other on this, as has the way the media have treated the issue, condemning social workers in one week for taking high-handed action in removing children from their families, and then condemning them for not taking action to protect a child the next week. In truth it is a dilemma as old as social work. There are other, similar dilemmas: whether to leave older people to face specific hazards (but of their choice), to release a person with severe mental health problems into the community, or to urge a person on incapacity benefit to get a job.

The lesson from history is this: the pendulum will not come to rest but will remain constantly in motion. It comes with the territory. Social scientists have looked at this phenomenon noting that there are specific practice contexts in which 'cycling or alternation' of policies and approaches is characteristic. This may arise from new visions of innovation 'often embarrassingly evangelical and unthought through', according to Pollitt (2008: 2), or because political cycles are short and politicians' expectations of their programmes likewise short. The culture of the social work organization is both a constraint from the past and a resource: expertise based on accumulating experience is preparation for the long term enabling social workers to deal with these perpetual dilemmas. To build this expertise, training professional staff to cope, individual motivation, values and attitudes are more important than formal systems (Pollitt 2008).

Gender

From the first, social work has been predominantly female, whether volunteer or paid organizer. (The exceptions are notable: NSPCC inspectors, school attendance officers, relieving officers in the days of the Poor Law, and mental welfare officers after the Second World War.) As discussed in Chapter 4, social work offered the prospect of involvement in public matters for middle-class women and, for some, professional attainment. As care responsibilities in the poor families with whom they worked also fell on women, gender became a central issue for social work on both sides of the worker/user divide. Whether in the COS or the settlement movement, psychiatric social workers (PSWs) within child guidance, moral welfare workers with unmarried mothers or as basic grade workers within the Seebohm departments, women have outnumbered men by a large proportion. The latest figures from the General Social Care Council indicate that 77 per cent of registered social workers – nearly eight out of ten – are women (GSCC 2011: 8). In Scotland, 85 per cent of social work services staff are female; for adult services the figure is over 89 per cent (Scottish Government 2011).

The question is a complex one: how does this gender imbalance affect social work and social workers? As Walkowitz has said, the social services workplace is a 'heterosocial one', creating problems for both men and women as their professional identity is tied to either masculinity or femininity (Walkowitz 1999: 12). For men, social work was a stepping-stone to a career in management. As he puts it: 'Women staked a claim to public space but discovered that men still ruled in it, men whose own masculinity depended on their dominance and higher wage' (ibid.: 12).

For women in social care there are what Nancy Folbre has called 'pink collar penalities': jobs that revolve around nurturance and caring are paid less than other lines of work, whereas jobs that involve exercising authority over other people are paid more (Folbre 2001). She imagines sarcastically what the conventional economist might say about this: 'That's the beauty of the market. Workers who provide care for other people get intrinsic satisfaction from doing those jobs, and that warm glow makes up the low pay. On the other hand, being a boss is *so* unpleasant – that's why the market rewards that kind of work more' (Folbre 2001: 45).

For users there must also be limitations. Social learning theory, the value of role modelling, use of self, shared experiences – all part of the social worker's repertoire – point to the value of a more gender-balanced occupation, particularly so, for example, in work with boys excluded from school or engaging in anti-social behaviour, or in work with fathers.

Interpreting social work history

While the mission of this volume has been to supply sufficient materials that readers can make up their own mind on the significance and direction of social work history, this final chapter does allow us to raise more directly the question, of whether there a single perspective or vantage point from which to understand a sizeable portion of what has happened. There are at least four plausible ways of understanding social work history: (i) what could be called the 'Whig' interpretation of history; (ii) Marxist perspectives on the development of social work; (iii) the development of social work as the result of professionalization; (iv) social work as a form of social control.

The 'Whig' interpretation of history

The Whigs were the precursors of the nineteenth-century Liberal Party – indeed they formed the government that passed the Poor Law Amendment Act of 1834. The notion of a 'Whig interpretation of history' derives from Herbert Butterfield's book of that title which took to task those who wrote history as a story of steady, continual progress towards the present (Butterfield 1931). This was best exemplified for Butterfield by the Whig/Liberal historians who charted British political history in those terms.'Whig' history became a byword for uncritical, essentially optimistic narratives in which all is for the best in the best of all possible worlds.

Social work has its own 'whiggish' versions in which each development in practice and the major pioneering individuals all add something of value to the narrative of steadily improving social work accomplishment. These are generally found among older accounts, for example in works by Bell (1961), Woodroofe (1962), Rooff (1972) and Seed (1973) in which continuous progress towards an ever more competent, contemporary profession unfolds. They are also found in short summaries of the origins of social work that sometimes introduce longer scholarly articles.

However, the development of social work was not, and certainly in the future will not be, a narrative in which it seamlessly improves upon itself. False steps and clashes between ideologies, social interests and social classes cannot be woven into a single uncritical narrative. Octavia Hill and the COS offer a perfect example. Many histories point to her involvement in establishing social work as a field of social practice but fold her and the COS into social work history without critical balance. Hill and the COS achieved much, but she also held ideas about work and poverty that were disputed even before the end of the nineteenth century. An account that places her in a seamless story of progress towards ever better versions of social work without acknowledging the repressive views she held regarding the urban working class cannot be a full account. Social work grew out from the evangelical impulses of the nineteenth century and the 'rage of Christian economics', as Boyd Hilton (1988) has put it – by which he means a zealous, fervent (and Protestant) attachment to the market, as the key to progress and the good society. Hill and the other prominent COS advocates picked up this mantle and put it on a better organized footing. But they remained wedded to the Poor Law system for decades. For example, some forty years after the founding of the COS and with many more complex explanations of urban poverty available, they not only dominated the Royal Commission on the Poor Laws and Relief of Distress that sat between 1905 and 1909 but one of their own, Helen Bosanquet, drafted a large part of the majority report of the Commission published in 1909. The public intellectuals of the COS were the original 'compassionate conservatives'; to their credit that compassion for the poor was authentic and deeply held, but they had long-standing total opposition to any state involvement in the relief of poverty outside the Poor Law system despite the weaknesses and limited scale of voluntary organizations that were already evident at the time. That we are heading back into an era of welfare policy based on a similar philosophy raises an interesting question: how will social work conduct itself this time around?

A similar point can be made in relation to mental welfare and mental deficiency: a sizeable swathe of social workers before and after the First World War held eugenicist views, and without an analysis of why it was so and its consequences, any history of social work is distorted. When Evelyn Fox set herself up in 1913 as the head of what later became the Central Association of Mental Welfare, she knew little about learning disability. What she advocated for the 'mentally deficient' – voluntary sterilization, segregation, surveillance – simply reflected the prejudice and sheer ignorance of the times. The reader looking for a good example of uncritical, whiggish-type history will find none better than the entry on Evelyn Fox in the *Oxford Dictionary of National Biography* (Thomas 2004), which does not mention her association with sterilization or eugenics.

Marxist interpretations

A classical Marxist interpretation of social work history would begin with the central idea that class conflict lies at the heart of all history, conflict between those who own the means of production (the bourgeoisie, or upper middle class, that either directly owns the means of production or possesses the capital to do so), and those who have to sell their labour power on the open market in order to survive – the working class. The interests of these two classes are antagonistic: the one exploits by extracting value over and above what it has to pay the worker, while the other resists that exploitation by drawing on power acquired through labour movement and trade union solidarity.

But after that starting point, Marxists might well develop differing accounts. One might consider social work as an arm of the bourgeoisie, inspecting, advising, pressuring working-class families to adhere to forms of work discipline and self-control that aid the functioning of production. Such an argument could have plausibility in relation to the practice of the COS – and in fact was widely held by the labour movement in the first part of the twentieth century – but would be more difficult to sustain as social work diversified, allying itself with policies of income support and wealth redistribution after the creation of the welfare state in 1945; and it would be harder still to square with the emergence of radical social work (itself often Marxist in orientation) in the 1970s.

A more nuanced interpretation, such as that by Peter Leonard (1979) moves beyond Marxist fundamentalism to argue that the Second World War showed the bourgeoisie the value of a healthy, reasonably educated and secure working class and therefore more receptive to establishing a welfare state. But Leonard also concludes that specific elements of the welfare state, such as the health service, national insurance and family allowance, were the result of years of working-class effort culminating in Labour's victory of 1945. He goes on to note that by the 1970s state-provided welfare had ossified, creating a purely 'client relationship' between the people and welfare services, one refusing to yield to calls for participation and democratization. It also involved the deskilling and bureaucratization of the welfare state's own employees as the state's search for efficiency led it to introduce corporate management techniques to 'replace the semi-autonomy of professional judgement with the reliability of the state functionary' (Leonard 1979).

In reference to the twenty-first century, Marxists might well note the near insoluble contradictions for social workers that the global economic crisis of 2008–09 has produced:

- The pressure on those outside the labour market, often service users – lone parents, those on incapacity benefit, young people without educational qualifications – to find work or lose benefits which had been theirs previously as of right.
- The squeeze on its own sources of employment along with the rest of the public sector as capital rationalizes its operations, by ensuring that the state takes as little from the pot of national wealth as possible.
- Extensive sell-off of public services to corporate interests and the hidden privatization of services as the personalization agenda slowly restricts the welfare state's capacity to pool risks and provide sufficiently resourced safety nets for all.
- The political context in which electorates across Europe, including Britain, have demonstrated a distrust both of large economic institutions and of the state, giving centre-right parties a free hand to replenish the main agents of the economic catastrophe – the banks – with huge flows of capital, while ensuring that those least responsible for the crisis – the public sector staff – are drained of funding.

A story of professional self-advancement

Another interpretation centres around social work as a self-promoting profession, what has been called the 'professionalisation of poverty' (Lowe and Reid

1999). In this critical account, social work sprang into being on the back of the notion that poverty was a consequence not of economic or social systems but of individual irresponsibility that needed correction and guidance. It is largely found in accounts of social work in the United States, such as those by Lubove (1969), Ehrenreich (1985) and Walkowitz (1999). Walkowitz's volume in particular superbly relates the growth of social work as a function of middle-class identity and an avenue enabling women to move into a profession; in the course of his narrative he supplies fine-grained analysis of what was taking place in particular agencies. Curiously, in Britain this interpretation of social work as means of professional advancement has thus far been absent.

Such an interpretation would focus on social work's long-term desire to become recognized as a fully fledged profession, which would then prompt questions about the real motivations behind social work claims for what it is able to achieve. As Ehrenreich (1985: 14) put it in relation to social work in the United States, social work has been 'obsessed with professional status'. It would also discuss the role of the professions and the way in which they have historically been able to restrict access into their ranks while at the same time ensuring that they were able to regulate themselves. But such an interpretation would no doubt have to conclude how this project was continually thwarted by a failure to define satisfactorily its domain of activity. Because of this social work could not establish borders that it could defend and within which it could assert its professional authority and drive out competitors. Finally it would have to reach some conclusion about the fact that social work is in essence a service for families on low income and high needs and that materially, whether in status or salaries, the rewards for such work are relatively low.

Social work as a form of social control

A fourth interpretation views social work as an agent of social control. Some follow Michel Foucault's conception – that power is embedded in everyday sources and institutions such as language, clinical conduct and psychiatric regimes. It is impossible to escape their 'gaze'; society is drenched in power (Foucault 1973). There is no history of social work in the UK that takes this view of power as its starting point; one has to look again to the United States for that. Margolin's *Under the Cover of Kindness* (1997) offers a persuasive account that sees each phase of social work's development as an expansion of power and influence over ever more disempowered users. In particular he describes the 'birth of the investigation', during the rise of the COS in the United States (directly transplanted from Britain), in which families had no means to shield from the investigators information they considered private and off limits. Every aspect of family life was of legitimate interest as far as the COS investigators were concerned. (Interestingly, the National Association of Social Workers in the United States warmly welcomed this highly critical account precisely because of its strong critical edge.) Nikolas Rose (1999), however, does offer an account of social policy in Britain based explicitly on Foucault in which he examines how various forms of psychological expertise and discourse have played a key role in the rationality of government and in the making up of governable subjects – children, citizens – 'and the kinds of legitimacy that they have accorded to those who want to exercise authority over human conduct' (Rose 1999: xxii).

However, many historians have come to view 'social control', with its implication that there is a centralized, hegemonic power governing all aspects of social life, as too simplistic an idea as it overlooks the continual process of negotiation, dispute and outright conflict that shapes policy in outcomes.

Yet the notion cannot be dismissed altogether in social work history. Indeed, understanding the informal means of establishing social control of particular groups of people is central to understanding that history. As we have seen, the surveillance and regulation of learning disabled people was the core task for social work in the first half of the twentieth century and beyond. So too was the oversight and control of other forms of behaviour – those with poor parenting skills, mental health problems, and drug and alcohol dependency. This responsibility lay with social work from its inception and continues to be a central feature, periodically generating profound enquiries into social work ethics and the use of power and authority.

Discussion point   If you had to choose one . . .

Of the four interpretations of social work history above, which one do you think would come closest to providing a coherent theory of social work history? Which one would you think was the least satisfactory?

Interpretations such as these can be helpful perspectives, throwing a spot light on one or other elements of social work's development. None however offers a once-for-all way of understanding that development. The future is open-ended and will produce contingencies, conflicts and practices that we can only guess at. Social work, as it must, will continue to change and adapt, and, as this history suggests, will, more than most other lines of professional practice, be responsive to the context and environment in which it works.

Bibliography

Abbott, P. and C. Wallace (1990). *The Sociology of the Caring Professions*. London: Falmer Press.

ADASS (Association of Directors of Adult Social Services) (2010). *The Future of Social Work in Adult Social Services in England*. London: ADASS/Department of Health. Available at http://www.dh.gov.uk/en/Publicationsandstatistics/Publications/PublicationsPolicyAndGuidance/DH_114571 (accessed 5 June 2011).

Agnew, E. (2004) *From Charity to Social Work: Mary E. Richmond and the Creation of an American Profession*. Urbana: University of Illinois Press.

Arnold, E., M. Bogle, et al. (1987). *Whose Child? The Report of the Public Inquiry into the Death of Tyra Henry*. London: London Borough of Lambeth.

Atkinson, D., M. Jackson and J. Walmsley (eds) (2000). *Good Times, Bad Times: Women with Learning Difficulties Telling their Stories*. Kidderminster: BILD.

Atkinson, D., M. Jackson and J. Walmsley (1997). *Forgotten Lives: Exploring the History of Learning Disability*. Kidderminster: BILD.

Atlee, C. (1920). *The Social Worker*. London: G. Bell & Sons.

Audit Commission (1986). *Making a Reality of Community Care*. London.

Bailey, R. and M. Brake (eds) (1975). *Radical Social Work*. London: Edward Arnold.

Bailey, V. (1987). *Deliquency and Citizenship: Reclaiming the Young Offender, 1914–1918*. Oxford: Clarendon Press.

Bain, A. (2004). 'From redemption to rehabilitation to resettlement', *Criminal Justice Matters* **56**(1): 8–10.

Bamford, T. (2001). *Commissioning and Purchasing*. London: Routledge.

Bamford, T. (1990). *The Future of Social Work*. Basingstoke: Macmillan.

Barber, J. (1991). *Beyond Casework*. London: Macmillan.

Barclay Committee (1982). *Social Workers: Their Role and Tasks* (Barclay Report). London: Bedford Square Press.

Bartlett, H. M. (1928). 'The social survey and the charity organization movement', *American Journal of Sociology* **34**(2): 330–46.

Bartley, P. (2000). *Prostitution: Prevention and Reform in England 1860–1914*. London: Routledge.

Batty, D. (2002) Q&A: The general social care council, www.guardian.co.uk/society/2002/jan/18/3 (accessed 12 February 2010).

Behlmer, G. K. (1998). *Friends of the Family: The English Home and its Guardians*. Stanford, CA: Stanford University Press.

Behlmer, G. K. (1982). *Child Abuse and Moral Reform in England 1870–1908*. Stanford, CA: Stanford University Press.

Bell, E. M. (1961). *The Story of Hospital Almoners: The Birth of a Profession*. London: Faber & Faber.

Beniger, J. (1986). *The Control Revolution: Technological and Economic Origins of the Information Society*. Cambridge, MA: Harvard University Press.

Benjamin, S. (2001). 'From "idiot child" to "mental defective": schooling and the production of intellectual disability in the UK 1850–1944', *Educate* **1**(1).

Berridge, V. (1990). 'Health and medicine', in F. M. L. Thompson (ed.) *The Cambridge Social History of Britain 1750–1950*. Cambridge: Cambridge University Press.

Besley, T. (2002). 'Social education and mental hygiene: Foucault, disciplinary technologies and the moral constitution of youth', *Educational Philosophy and Theory* **34**(4): 419–33.

Beveridge, W. (1942). *Report of the Inter-Departmental Committee on Social Insurance and Allied Service* (Beveridge Report), Cmnd 6404. London: HMSO.

Beveridge, W. and A. Wells (1949). *The Evidence for Voluntary Action: being memoranda by organisations and individuals and other material relevant to voluntary action*. London: Allen & Unwin.

Biestek, F. (1961). *The Casework Relationship*. London: George Allen & Unwin.

Bilton, K. (2011). 'Fighting for the identity of social work', Social Work History Network seminar, University College London, 20 May.

Birt, L. (1913). *The Children's Home-Finder: The Story of Annie MaPherson and Louise Birt*. London: James Nisbet & Co.

Bissell, V. (2007). *The Education of Jane Addams*. Philadelphia: University of Pennsylvania Press.

Booth, C. (1903). *Life and Labour of the People in London*, 3rd edn, vol. 3. London.

Booth, C. (1893). *Life and Labour of the People of London*, vol. 4: *Religious Life*. London: Macmillan & Co.

Bosanquet, B. (1907). *The Social Criterion Or, How to Judge Proposed Social Reforms*. Edinburgh: William Blackwood & Sons.

Bosanquet, B. (1901). 'The meaning of social work', *International Journal of Ethics* **11**: 291.

Bosanquet, B. (1895). 'The duties of citizenship', in Bosanquet (ed.) *Aspects of the Social Problem*. London: Macmillan & Co.

Bosanquet, B. (1874). *The Organisation of Charity: The History and Mode of Operation of the Charity Organisation Society*. London: Longmans, Green & Co.

Bosanquet, H. (1914). *Social Work in London 1869–1912: A History of the Charity Organisation Society*. London: John Murray.

Bosanquet, H. (1903). *The Strength of the People: A Study in Social Economics*. London: Macmillan.

Braithwaite, E. (1962). *Paid Servant*. London: The Bodley Head.

Braye, S. (2000). 'Participation and involvement in social care: an overview', in H. Kemshall and R. Littlechild (eds) *User Involvement and Participation in Social Care*. London: Jessica Kingsley Publishers.

Braye, S. and M. Preston-Shoot (1995). *Empowering Practice in Social Care*. Buckingham: Open University Press.

Brewer, C. and J. Lait (1980). *Can Social Work Survive?* London: Maurice Temple Smith.

Briggs, A. and A. Macartney (1984). *Toynbee Hall: The First Hundred Years*. London: Routledge & Kegan Paul.

Brill, K. and R. Thomas (1964). *Children in Homes*. London: Gollancz.

Brock, L. G. (1931). 'Mental health workers: an appreciation', *Mental Welfare* **12**.

Bulmer, M. and J. Bulmer (1981). 'Philanthropy and social science in the 1920s: Beardsley Ruml and the Laura Spellman Rockefeller Memorial 1922–29', *Minerva* **19**(3): 347–407.

Burnett, R. and C. Appleton (2004). Joined-Up Services To Tackle Youth Crime: A Case Study in England, *British Journal of Criminology* **44**: 34–54.

Burt, C. (1925). *The Young Delinquent*. London: University of London Press.

Butler-Sloss, L. (1988). *Report of the Inquiry into Child Abuse in Cleveland 1987*. London: HMSO.

Butterfield, H. (1931). *The Whig Interpretation of History*. London: George Bell & Sons.

Cahill, M. and T. Jowitt (1980). 'The new philanthropy: the emergence of the Bradford Guild of Help', *Journal of Social Policy* **9**: 359–82.

Cavenagh, W. E. (1956). *Four Decades of Students in Social Work*. Birmingham: University of Birmingham.

Cawthorn, C. (2010). Conversation with Craig Cawthorn.

Cawthorn, C. (2011). Conversation with Craig Cawthorn.

CCETSW (Central Council for Education and Training in Social Work) (1991). *Rules and Requirements for the Diploma in Social Work* (Paper 30). London: CCETSW.

Chaplin, C. (1964). *My Autobiography*. London: Penguin.

Charity Organisation Society (1939). 'Family casework and mental health', *Charity Organisation Quarterly* **13**: 40–50.

Clarke, J. (1971). 'An analysis of crisis management by mental welfare officers', *British Journal of Social Work* **1**(1): 27–38.

Clarke Hall, W. (1926). *Children's Courts*. London: Allen & Unwin.

Clement Brown, S. (1939). 'The methods of social case workers', in F. Bartlett, M. Ginsburg, E. Lindgren and R. Thouless (eds) *The Study of Society*. London: Kegan Paul, Trench, Trubner & Co.

Clough, R. (1999). 'Scandalous care: interpreting public enquiry reports of scandals in residential care', *Elder Abuse and Neglect in Residential Settings* **10**(1/2): 13–27.

Clyde, J. (1946). *Report of the Committee on Homeless Children*, Cmnd 6911. Edinburgh: HMSO.

Community Care (1982). News: 'Approved social workers', August 12.

Community Care (2003). News: 'Everybody Out', 10 July.

Cooper, J. (1983). *Creation of the British Personal Social Services 1962–1974*. London: Heinemann.

Corby, B. (1987). *Working with Child Abuse.* Milton Keynes: Open University Press.

Corrigan, P. and P. Leonard (1978). *Social Work Practice under Capitalism: A Marxist Approach.* London: Macmillan.

Cree, V. (1992). 'Social work's changing task: an analysis of the changing task of social workers seen through the history and development of one Scottish organisation, Family Care', PhD thesis, University of Edinburgh.

Cretney, S. (2004). *Family Law in the Twentieth Century: A History.* Oxford: Oxford University Press.

Crocker, R. H. (1992). *Social Work and Social Order: The Settlement Movement in Industrial Cities 1889–1930.* Urbana: University of Illinois Press.

Cullen, L. (2009). 'The first lady almoner: the appointment, position and findings of Miss Mary Stewart at the Royal Free Hospital 1895–1899', Seminar, Institute of Historical Research, 28 September.

Curtis, M. (1946) *Report of the Care of Children Committee* (Curtis Report), Cmnd 6922. London: HMSO.

Dale, P. (2006). 'Tension in the voluntary–statutory alliance: "lay professionals" and the planning and delivery of mental deficiency services 1917–45', in P. Dale and J. Melling (eds) *Mental Illness and Learning Disability since 1850: Finding a Place for Mental Disorder in the United Kingdom.* Abingdon: Routledge.

Darley, G. (1990). *Octavia Hill.* London: Constable.

Daunton, M., (ed.) (2000). *The Cambridge Urban History of Britain.* Cambridge: Cambridge University Press.

Daunton, M. (1996). 'Welfare and state formation in Britain 1900–1951', *Past and Present* **150**: 169–216.

Davies, B. (1992). *Care Management: Equity and Efficiency, The International Experience.* Canterbury: Personal Social Services Research Unit, University of Kent.

Davies, M. (1981). *The Essential Social Worker: A Guide to Positive Practice.* London: Heinemann Education and Community Care.

Department of Health (2007). *Putting People First.* London: Department of Health.

Department of Health (2006). *Our Health, Our Care, Our Say: A New Direction for Community Services.* London: Department of Health.

Department of Health (2003). *Fair Access to Care Services: Guidance on Eligibility Criteria for Adult Social Care.* London: Department of Health.

Department of Health (2000a). *Assessment of Children in Need.* London: The Stationery Office.

Department of Health (2000b). *A Quality Strategy for Social Care.* London: Department of Health.

Department of Health (1998). *Modernising Social Services: Promoting Independence, Improving Protection, Raising Standards,* Cm 4169. London: The Stationery Office.

Department of Health (1991). *Care Management and Assessment: Practitioners' Guide.* London: Department of Health, Social Services Inspectorate/Scottish Office, Social Work Services Group.

Department of Health (1990). *Community Care in the Next Decade and Beyond.* London: HMSO.

Department of Health and Social Security (1980) *Child Abuse: Central Register Systems,* LASSL (80) 4: HN (80) 20.

Department of Health and Social Security (1974). *Non-Accidental Injury to Children,* LASSL (74) 13. London.

Digby, A. (1996). 'Contexts and perspectives', in D. Wright and A. Digby (eds) *From Idiocy to Mental Deficiency: Historical Perspectives on People with Learning Difficulties.* London: Routledge.

Dominelli, L. (1996). 'Deprofessionalizing social work: anti-oppressive practice, competencies and postmodernism', *British Journal of Social Work* **26**(2): 153–75.

Donnison, D., P. Jay and M. Stewart (1962). *The Ingleby Report: Three Critical Essays.* London: The Fabian Society.

Dumsday W. and J. Moss (1929). *The Relieving Officers' Handbook* 4th ed London: Hadden, Best and Co. Ltd.

Dunleavy, P. and C. Hood (1994). 'From old public administration to new public management', *Public Money and Management* **14**(3): 9–16.

Eaton, L. (1994). 'Why is community care failing the mentally ill?' *Community Care,* Reed Business Publishing, pp. 7–9.

Ehrenreich, J. H. (1985). *The Altruistic Imagination: A History of Social Work and Social Policy in the United States.* Ithaca, NY: Cornell University Press.

Ellis, K., A. Davis and K. Rummery (1999). 'Needs assessment, street-level bureaucracy and the new community care', *Social Policy and Administration* **33**(3): 262–80.

Etzioni, A. (1969). *Semi-Professions and their Organizations: Teachers, Nurses, Social Workers.* New York: The Free Press.

Family Rights Group (1986). *Promoting Links: Keeping Children and Families in Touch.* London: Family Rights Group.

Ferguson, H. (2003). 'Protecting children in new times: child protection and the risk society', *Child and Family Social Work* **2**(4): 221–34.

Ferguson, S. and H. Fitzgerald (1954). *Studies in the Social Services: History of the Second World War.* London: HMSO.

Finer, M. (1974). *Report of the Committee on One-Parent Families* (Finer Report), Cmnd 5629. London: Department of Health and Social Security.

Finkelstein, V. (1975). *UPIAS Principles: Fundamental Principles of Disability.* London: UPIAS. Available at www.leeds.ac.uk/disability-studies/.../fundamental%20principles.pdf.

Finlayson, G. (1994). *Citizen, State, and Social Welfare in Britain 1830–1990.* Oxford: Clarendon Press.

Fisher, T. (1974). *Committee of Inquiry into the Care and Supervision Provided in Relation to Maria Colwell* London: HMSO.

Flexner, A. (1915). 'Is social work a profession?' Paper presented at the National Conference on Charities and Correction, Baltimore, MD, Proceedings, pp. 581–90.

Folbre, N. (2001). *The Invisible Heart: Economics and Family Values*. New York: New Press.

Foucault, M. (1973). *The Birth of the Clinic*. London: Tavistock.

Fox, E. (1938). 'Modern developments in mental welfare work', *Eugenics Review* **30**(3): 165–73.

Fox, E. (1929) *CAMW Conference Report*, Central Association of Mental Welfare.

Freeden, M. (1979). 'Eugenics and progressive thought: a study in ideological affinity', *History Journal* **22**: 645–71.

Frere, M. (1909). *Children's Care Committees*. London: P.S. King & Son.

Friedson, E. (1970). *Profession of Medicine: A Study of the Sociology of Applied Knowledge*. Chicago: University of Chicago Press.

Furgol, M. T. (1987). 'Thomas Chalmers's poor relief theories and their implementation', PhD thesis, Edinburgh University.

Gabriel, J. M. (2005). 'Mass producing the individual: Mary C. Jarret, Elmer E. Southard, and the industrial origins of psychiatric social work', *Bulletin of the History of Medicine* **79**(3): 430–58.

GSCC (2011). *Annual Report and Accounts 2009–2010*. London: General Social Care Council.

Gente, M. (2002). 'Family ideology and the Charity Organization in Great Britain during the First World War', *Journal of Family History* **27**(3): 255–72.

Gilbert, B. (1966). *The Evolution of National Insurance in Great Britain: The Origin of the Welfare State*. London: Michael Joseph.

Glasby, J. (2000). *'Back to the Future': The History of the Settlement Movement*. Birmingham: Birmingham University.

Glover-Thomas, N. (2002). *Reconstructing Mental Health Law and Policy*. London: Butterworths.

Glueck, B. (1934). 'Child guidance', *Encyclopedia of the Social Sciences*. New York: Macmillan.

Goffman, E. (1961). *Asylums: Essays on the Social Situation of Mental Patients and other Inmates*. London: Pelican.

Goldstein, J., A. Freud and A. Solnit (1973). *Beyond the Best Interests of the Child*. Boston: The Free Press.

Goodlad, L. (2001). ' "Making the working man like me": charity, pastorship, and middle-class identity in nineteenth-century Britain; Thomas Chalmers and Dr. James Phillips Kay', *Victorian Studies* **43**(4): 591–617.

Gostin, L. (1984). 'The Mental Health Act', *Social Work Today*, 5 November.

Gostin, L. (1975). *A Human Condition*. London: MIND.

Griffiths, R. (1988) *Community Care: Agenda for Action* (Griffiths Report). London: HMSO.

Hadley, R., M. Cooper, P. Dale and G. Stacy (1987). *A Community Social Worker's Handbook*. London: Tavistock.

Hall, P. (1976). *Reforming the Welfare: The Politics of Change in the Personal Social Services*. London: Heinemann.

Hall, P., H. Land, et al. (1975). *Change, Choice and Conflict in Social Policy*. London: Heinemann.

Hancock Nunn, T. (1914). 'Councils of Social Service', *Charity Organisation Review* **36**: 58–62.

Handler, J. (1973). *The Coercive Social Worker: British Lessons for American Social Services*. Chicago: Rand McNally.

Hanvey, C. (2011). 'Fighting for the identity of social work: a historical perspective on the idea of a social work college', Social Work History Network seminar, University College London, 20 May.

Hardiker, P. and M. Barker (1981). *Theories of Practice in Social Work*. London: Academic Press.

Harris, John (2003). *The Social Work Business*. London: Routledge.

Harris, Jose (1992). 'Political thought and the welfare state 1870–1940: an intellectual framework for British social policy', *Past and Present* **135**: 116–41.

Harrison, B. (1976). 'Miss Butler's Oxford Survey', in A. Halsey (ed.) *Traditions of Social Policy: Essays in Honour of Violet Butler*. Oxford: Basil Blackwell.

Hatfield, B. (2008). 'Powers to detain under mental health legislation in England and the role of the approved social worker: an analysis of patterns and trends under the 1983 Mental Health Act in six local authorities', *British Journal of Social Work* **38**: 1553–71.

Heeny, B. (1983). 'Women's struggle for professional work and status in the Church of England 1900–1930', *The Historical Journal* **26**(2): 329–47.

Hendrick, H. (1994). *Child Welfare in England 1872–1989*. London: Routledge.

Heywood, J. (1978). *Children in Care*. London: Routledge.

Hill, M. (ed.) (2000). *Local Authority Social Services: An Introduction*. Oxford: Blackwell.

Hill, O. (1875). *Homes of the London Poor*. London: Macmillan.

Hill, O. (2010 [1875]). *Our Common Land*. Cambridge: Cambridge University Press.

Hill, O. (1872, various). *Letters to Fellow Workers*. London: Institute of Economic Affairs.

Hilton, B. (1988). *The Age of Atonement: The Influence of Evangelicalism on Social and Economic Thought, 1795–1865*. Oxford: Clarendon Press.

Himmelfarb, G. (1992). *Poverty and Compassion: The Moral Imagination of the Late Victorians*. New York: Vintage Books.

Hobhouse, R. W. (1913). *The Life of Benjamin Waugh*. London: T.F. Unwin.

Hobsbawm, E. (1988). *The Age of Revolution*. London: Abacus.

Hobson, J. (1909). *The Crisis of Liberalism: New Issues of Democracy*. London: King Publishing.

Holman, B. (2001). *Champions for Children: The Lives of Modern Child Care Pioneers*. Cambridge: Polity Press.

Holman, B. (1996). *The Corporate Parent: Manchester Children's Department 1948–1971*. London: National Institute for Social Work.

Holman, B. (1995). *The Evacuation: A Very British Revolution*. Oxford: Lion Publishing.

Home Office (1933). Circular 9, *Children and Young Persons Act 1933*. London.

Hopkinson, A. (1976). *Single Mothers: The First Year*. Edinburgh: Scottish Council for Single Parents.

Hoppen, T. (1998). *The Mid-Victorian Generation 1846–1886*. Oxford: Clarendon Press.

House of Commons Committee on Children, Schools and Families (2009). *Third Report: Looked-after Children* Chapter 2 www.publications.parliament.uk/pa/cm200809/cmselect/cmchilsch/111/1110/6.htm (accessed 24 February 2011).

Howard, A. (ed.) (1979). *The Crossman Diaries: Selections from the Diaries of a Cabinet Minister 1964–1970*. London: Magnum Books.

Howe, D. (2008). 'Child abuse and the bureaucratisation of social work', *Sociological Review* **40**(3): 491–508.

Hugman, R. (2003). 'Religious dimensions of the origins of professional social work and the possibility of an international code of ethics', *Professional Ethics* **11**(1): 37–54.

Humphreys, R. (1995). *Sin, Organised Charity and the Poor Law in Victorian England*. London: St Martin's Press.

Hunnybun, N. (1950). 'Psychiatric social work', in C. Morris (ed.) *Social Case-work in Great Britain*. London: Faber & Faber.

Hyland, J. (2009). *Changing Times, Changing Needs*. London: Catholic Children's Society (Westminster).

Illich, I. (1975). 'Clinical damage, medical monopoly, the expropriation of health: three dimensions of iatrogenic tort', *Journal of Medical Ethics* **1**: 78–80.

Ingleby Committee (1960). *Report of the Committee on Children and Young Persons*, Cmnd 1191. London: HMSO.

Jackson, M. (2004). 'Dendy, Mary (1855–1933)', *Oxford Dictionary of National Biography*. Oxford: Oxford University Press. Available at http://www.oxforddnb.com/view/article/51775 (accessed 6 July 2011).

Jackson, S. (1998). 'Educational success for looked after children: the social worker's responsibility', *Practice* **10**(4): 47–56.

Jarrett, M. (1921). 'The practical value of mental hygiene in industry', *Hospital Social Services* **3**: 361–5.

Jennings, H. (1930). *The Private Citizen in Public Social Work*. London: Allen & Unwin.

JM Consulting (1999). *Review of the Diploma in Social Work*. Bristol: JM Consulting Ltd.

Jones, C. (2001). 'Voices from the front line: state social workers and New Labour', *British Journal of Social Work* **31**(4): 547–62.

Jones, K. (2000). *The Making of Social Policy in Britain: From Poor Law to New Labour*. London: The Athlone Press.

Jones, K. (1993). *Asylums and After: A Revised History of the Mental Health Services from the Early 18th Century to the 1990s*. London: The Athlone Press.

Jones, K. (ed.) (1972). *The Year Book of Social Policy, 1971*. London: Routledge.

Jordan, B. (2004). 'Emancipatory social work: opportunity or oxymoron?' *British Journal of Social Work* **34**(1): 5–19.

Keating, J. (2008). *A Child for Keeps: The History of Adoption in England 1918–1945*. Basingstoke: Palgrave Macmillan.

Keating, J. (2001). 'Struggle for identity: issues underlying the enactment of the 1926 Adoption of Children Act', *University of Sussex Journal of Contemporary History* **3**.

Kellogg, P. and A. Gleason (1919). *British Labor and the War*. New York: Boni & Liveright.

Kemshall, H., N. Parton, M. Walsh and E. J. Waterson (1997). 'Concepts of risk as core influences on organisational structure and functioning within the personal social services and Probation', *Social Policy and Administration* **31**: 213–32.

Kendall, K. A. (2000). *Social Work Education: Its Origins in Europe*. Alexandria, VA: Council of Social Work Education.

Kilbrandon Committee (1964) *Children and Young Persons, Scotland* (Kilbrandon Report), Cmnd 2306. Edinburgh: HMSO. Available at www.scotland.gov. uk/Publications/2003/10/18259/26883 (accessed 28 November 2010).

King, D. and R. Hansen (1999). 'Experts at work: state autonomy, social learning and eugenic sterilization in the 1930s', *British Journal of Political Science* **29**: 77–107.

King, M. (1995). 'The James Bulger murder trial: moral dilemmas, and social solutions', *International Journal of Children's Rights* **3**: 167–87.

Kunitz, S. (1974). 'Professionalism and social control in the progressive era: the case of the Flexner Report', *Social Problems* **22**(1): 16–27.

Laming, Lord (2003). *The Victoria Climbié Inquiry: Report of an Inquiry by Lord Laming*, Cm 5730. London: HMSO.

Law Commission (2011). *Adult Social Care: Summary of Final Report*, www. justice.gov.uk/lawcommission/adult-social-care.htm (accessed 23 May 2011).

LCC (1936). *Handbook on Mental Health Social Work*. London: Public Health Department, London County Council.

Leadbetter, C. (2004). *Personalisation*. London: Demos.

Lee, P. and M. Kenworthy (1928). *Mental Hygiene and Social Work*. New York: The Commonwealth Fund.

Lees, R. (1971). 'Social work 1925–1950: the case for reappraisal', *British Journal of Social Work* **1**: 371–9.

Leighton, B. (ed.) (1872). *Letters and other Writings of the late Edward Denison, M.P. for Newark*. London: Bentley & Son.

Leonard, P. (1979). 'Restructuring the welfare state', *Marxism Today*, December, pp. 7–13.

Leonard, P. (ed.) (1975). *The Sociology of Community Action*, Sociological Review Monograph. Hanley, Stoke on Trent: University of Keele.

Levy, A. and B. Kahan (1991). *The Pindown Experience and the Protection of Children: The Report of the Staffordshire Care Inquiry*. Staffordshire County Council.

Lewis, J. (1995a). 'Family provision of health and welfare in the mixed economy of care in the late nineteenth and twentieth centuries', *Society for the Social History of Medicine* **8**(1): 1–16.

Lewis, J. (1995b). *The Voluntary Sector, the State and Social Work in Britain: The Charity Organisation Society/Family Welfare Association since 1869*. Aldershot: Edward Elgar.

Lewis, J. (1980). *The Politics of Motherhood: Child and Maternal Welfare in England, 1900–1939*. London: Croom Helm.

Liddon, H. (1873). *Penitentiary Work in the Church of England*. London: Council of the Church Penitentiary Association.

Lloyd, L. (2006) 'The ethics of care and social work with older people', *British Journal of Social Work* **36**: 1171–85.

Loch, C. S. (1910). *Charity and Social Life: A Short Study of Religious and Social Thought in relation to Charitable Methods and Institutions*. London: Macmillan & Co.

Long, V. (2006). '"A satisfactory job is the best psychotherapist": employment and mental health, 1939–60', in J. Melling and P. Dale (eds) *Mental Illness and Learning Disability since 1850: Finding a Place for Mental Disorder in the United Kingdom*. Abingdon: Routledge.

Lowe, G. R. and P. N. Reid (eds) (1999). *The Professionalization of Poverty: Social Work and the Poor in the Twentieth Century*. New York: Aldine De Gruyter.

Lowe, R. (1986). *Adjusting to Democracy: The Role of the Ministry of Labour in British Politics 1916–1939*. Oxford: Clarendon Press.

Lubove, R. (1969). *The Professional Altruist: The Emergence of Social Work as a Career 1880–1930*. New York: Atheneum.

Lymbery, M. (2001). 'Social work at the crossroads', *British Journal of Social Work* **31**: 369–84.

Lymbery, M. (1998). 'Care management and professional autonomy: the impact of community care legislation on social work with older people', *British Journal of Social Work* **28**(6): 863–78.

Macadam, E. (1934). *The New Philanthropy*. London: Allen & Unwin.

Macadam, E. (1925). *The Equipment of the Social Worker*. London: George Allen & Unwin.

Mackintosh, J. M. (1951). *Report of the Committee on Social Workers in the Mental Health Services* (Mackintosh Report), Cmnd 8260. London: HMSO.

Macnicol, J. (1981). *The Movement for Family Allowance 1918–1945*. London: Heinemann.

Macpherson, W. (1999). *The Stephen Lawrence Inquiry*, Cm 4262-I. London: The Stationery Office.

Manthorpe, J. (2002). 'Settlements and social work education: absorption and accomodation', *Social Work Education* **21**(4): 410–19.

Margolin, L. (1997). *Under the Cover of Kindness: The Invention of Social Work*. Charlottesville: University of Virginia Press.

Marshall, M. (1983). *Social Work with Old People*. London: British Association of Social Workers and the Macmillan Press.

Martin, K. (2008). *Hard and Unreal Advice: Mothers, Social Science and Victorian Poverty Experts*. Basingstoke: Palgrave Macmillan.

Mayhew, B. (2006). 'Between love and aggression: the politics of John Bowlby', *History of the Human Sciences* **19**(4): 19–35.

McDougall, K. and U. Cormack (1950). 'Case-work in practice' in C. Morris (ed.) *Social Case-Work in Great Britain*. London: Faber & Faber.

McGhee, J., L. Waterhouse and B. Whyte (1996). 'Children's hearings and children in trouble', in S. Asquith (ed.) *Children and Young People in Conflict with the Law*. London: Jessica Kingsley Publishers.

Meacham, S. (1987). *Toynbee Hall and Social Reform 1880–1914: The Search for Community*. New Haven, CT: Yale University Press.

Mearns, A. (1970[1883]). *The Bitter Cry of Outcast London*. Leicester: Leicester University Press.

Millet, S. (1995). 'The age of criminal responsibility in an era of violence: has Great Britain set a new international standard?' *Vanderbilt Journal of Transnational Law* **28**: 295–347.

Millham, S., R. Bullock, et al. (eds) (1986). *Lost in Care: The Problems of Maintaining Links between Children in Care and their Families*. Aldershot: Gower.

Mills, C. W. (1943). 'The professional ideology of social pathologists', *American Journal of Sociology* **49**: 165–80.

Ministry of Health (1943). *The Break Up of the Poor Law and the Care of Children and Old People*. London.

Monckton, W. (1945). *Report on the circumstances which led to the boarding out of Dennis and Terrence O'Neill at Bank Farm, Minsterly and the steps taken to supervise their welfare* London: Home Office.

Moore, M. J. (1977). 'Social work and social welfare: the organization of philanthropic resources in Britain, 1900–1914', *Journal of British Studies* **16**: 85–104.

Moorehouse, W. (1911). Speech to Board of guardians www.meanwoodpark hospital.pikfu.net/set1635728/ (accessed March 3 2011).

Morris, C. (ed.) (1950). *Social Case-Work in Great Britain*. London: Faber & Faber.

Morris, P. (1984). 'Birmingham faces "biggest changes for ten years"', *Community Care* February 23 Business Press International, p. 5.

Morrison, W. (1998). 'Traditional values, children's rights and social justice: English youth justice in the 1990s', in G. Douglas and L. Sebba (eds) *Children's Rights and Traditional Values*. Aldershot: Ashgate.

Munro, E. and M. Calder (2005). 'Where has child protection gone?' *Political Quarterly* **76**(3): 439–45.

Munro, E. (1999). 'Common errors of reasoning in child protection work', *Child Abuse and Neglect* **23**(8): 745–58.

Murphy. J. (1992). *British Social Services: The Scottish Dimension*. Edinburgh: Scottish Academic Press.

Neill, J., I. Sinclair and P. Gorbach (1986). *Criteria for Part III Care: Report to the DHSS*. London: National Institute for Social Work.

NISW (National Institute for Social Work) (1988). *Residential Care for Elderly People: Using Research to Improve Practice*. London: National Institute for Social Work.

Oliver, M. (1989). 'Disability and dependency: a creation of industrial societies?' in L. Barton (ed.) *Disability and Dependency*. London: Falmer Press.

Oliver, M. (1984). *Social Work with Disabled People*. London: Macmillan.

Orme, J. (2001). 'Regulation or fragmentation? Directions for social work under New Labour', *British Journal of Social Work* **31**: 611–24.

Packman, J. (1975). *The Child's Generation: Child Care Policy from Curtis to Houghton*. Oxford: Basil Blackwell.

Page, R. and R. Silburn (1999). *British Social Welfare in the Twentieth Century*. Basingstoke: Macmillan.

Pankhurst, E. (1985[1914]). *My Own Story*. London: Greenwood Press.

Parker, J. (1965). *Local Health and Welfare Services*. London: Allen & Unwin.

Parker, R. (1966). *Decision in Child Care*. London: Allen & Unwin.

Parry, N., M. Rustin and C. Satyamurti (eds) (1979). *Social Work, Welfare and the State*. London: Edward Arnold.

Parton, N. (1979). 'The natural history of child abuse: a study in social problem definition', *British Journal of Social Work* **9**: 431–51.

Payne, M. (2005). *The Origins of Social Work: Community and Change*. London: Palgrave Macmillan.

Payne, M. (2002). 'The role and achievements of a professional association in the late twentieth century: the British Association of Social Workers 1970–2000', *British Journal of Social Work* **32**: 969–95.

Payne, S. (1999). 'Outside the walls of the asylum? Psychiatric treatment in the 1980s and 1990s', in P. Bartlett and D. Wright (eds) *Outside the Walls of the Asylum: The History of Community Care 1750–2000*. London: The Athlone Press.

Pearson, G. (1973). 'Social work as the privatised solution to public ills', *British Journal of Social Work* **3**(2): 209–23.

Penketh, L. (2000). *Tackling Institutional Racism: Anti-Racist Policies and Social Work Education and Training*. Bristol: Policy Press.

Perkin, H. (1989). *The Rise of Professional Society: England since 1880*. London: Routledge.

Perlman, H. (1957). *Social Casework: A Problem Solving Process*. Chicago: University of Chicago Press.

Philpot, T. (2000). Obituary: Barbara Kahan, *The Guardian*, 9 August.

Philpot, T. (1994) *Action for Children: The Story of Britain's Foremost Children's Charity*. Oxford: Lion Publishing.

Philpot, T. (1977). 'Crossman: his part in your service', *Community Care*, Reed International, pp. 15–16.

Philpot, T. (1991). The professional press: social work talking to itself, in B. Franklin and N. Parton (eds.) *Social Work, the Media and Public Relations*. London: Routledge.

Pierson, J. (1999). 'The mixed legacy of radical anti-oppressive practice', in T. Philpot (ed.) *Political Correctness and Social Work*. London: Institute of Economic Affairs.

Pimlott, J. A. R. (1935). *Toynbee Hall, Fifty Years of Social Progress 1884–1934*. London: J.M. Dent & Sons.

Pinker, R. (1993). 'A lethal kind of looniness', *Times Higher Education Supplement*, 10 September.

Pinker, R. (1982). 'An alternative view', in Barclay Committee Report, *Social Workers: Their Role and Tasks*. London: Bedford Square Press.

Plant, R. (1970). *Social and Moral Theory in Casework*. London: Routledge & Kegan Paul.

Pollitt, C. (2008). *Time, Policy, Management: Governing with the Past*. Oxford: Oxford University Press.

Poor Law Board (1870). *Orders and Regulations of the Poor Law Board for the Boarding Out of Pauper Children*. London: Shaw.

Postle (2001). 'The social work side is disappearing. I guess it started with us being called care managers', *Practice* **13**(1): 13–26.

Pringle, J. (1928). 'Impressions of a visit to the North American C.O.S.', *Charity Organisation Quarterly* (40–44).

Prior, P. (1992). 'The approved social worker: reflections on origins', *British Journal of Social Work* **22**: 105–19.

Prochaska, F. (2006). *Christianity and Social Service in Modern Britain: The Disinherited Spirit*. Oxford: Oxford University Press.

Rathbone, E. (1924). *The Disinherited Family*. London: Edward Arnold.

Reid, W. and L. Epstein (1972). *Task Centered Casework*. New York: Columbia University Press.

Reid, W. and A. W. Shyne (1969). *Brief and Extended Casework*. New York: Columbia University Press.

Richmond, M. E. (1917). *Social Diagnosis*. New York: Russell Sage Foundation.

Rimmer, J. (1980). *Troubles Shared: The Story of a Settlement 1899–1979*. Birmingham: Phlogiston Publishing.

Roberts, M. (1991) 'Reshaping the gift relationship: the London Mendicity Society and the suppression of begging in England 1818–1869', *International Journal of Social History* **36**: 201–31.

Roberts, M. J. D. (2004). *Making English Morals: Voluntary Association and Moral Reform in England, 1787–1886*. Cambridge: Cambridge University Press.

Robinson, V. (1930). *A Changing Psychology in Social Case Work*. Chapel Hill: University of North Carolina Press.

Rodgers, D. (1998). *Atlantic Crossings: Social Politics in a Progressive Age*. Cambridge, MA: The Belknap Press of Harvard University Press.

Rogowski, S. (2010). *Social Work The Rise and Fall of a Profession?* Bristol: Policy Press.

Rolph, S., D. Atkinson and J. Walmsley (2003). '"A pair of stout shoes and an umbrella": The role of the mental welfare officer in delivery community care in East Anglia, 1946–1970', *British Journal of Social Work* **33**: 339–59.

Rooff, M. (1972). *A Hundred Years of Family Welfare: A Study of the Family Welfare Association (formerly Charity Organisation Society 1869–1969)*. London: Michael Joseph.

Rooff, M. (1957). *Voluntary Society and Social Policy*. London: Routledge & Kegan Paul.

Rose, N. (1999). *Governing the Soul: The Shaping of the Private Self*, 2nd edn. London: Free Association Books.

Ross, E. (1993). *Love and Toil: Motherhood in Outcast London 1870–1918*. Oxford: Oxford University Press.

Rowe, J. and L. Lambert (1973). *Children Who Wait: A Study of Children Needing Substitute Families*. London: Association of British Adoption Agencies.

Rowntree, S. (1901). *Poverty: A Study of Town Life*. London: Macmillan.

Rummery, K. and C. Glendinning (1999) 'Negotiating needs, access and gatekeeping: developments in health and community care policies in the UK and the rights of disabled and older citizens', *Critical Social Policy* **19**(3): 335–51.

Sainsbury, E. (1970). *Social Diagnosis in Casework*. London: Routledge & Kegan Paul.

Satyamurti, C. (1981). *Occupational Survival*. Oxford: Basil Blackwell.

Sayce, L. (1994). 'An alternative view', *Community Care* (Supplement), Reed Business Publishing, pp. 9–11.

Scarman, Lord (1982) *The Brixton Disorders: The Scarman Report*. London: Penguin Books.

Schafer, A. (2002). 'Britain, Europe and the critique of capitalism in American reform 1880–1920', in M. Bever and F. Trentman (eds) *The Critique of Capitalism in American Reform 1880–1920*. Basingstoke: Palgrave Macmillan.

Schama, S. (2010). 'My vision for history in schools', *The Guardian*, 9 November.

Schön, D. (1983). *The Reflective Practitioner: How Professionals Think in Action*. London: Temple Smith.

Schur, E. M. (1973). *Radical Nonintervention: Rethinking the Delinquency Problem*. Englewood Cliffs, NJ: Prentice-Hall.

Scottish Government (2011). *Social Work Services Staff: Workforce by Client Group and Gender*, http://www.scotland.gov.uk/Topics/Statistics/Browse/Children/ TrendWorkforceGroupGender (accessed 20 May 2011).

Scull, A. T. (1989). *Social Order, Mental Disorder: Anglo-American Psychiatry in Historical Perspective*. London: Routledge.

Scull, A. T. (1982). *Museums of Madness: The Social Organization of Insanity in 19th Century England*. Harmondsworth: Penguin.

Seed, P. (1973). *The Expansion of Social Work in Britain*. London: Routledge & Kegan Paul.

SIAG (Seebohm Implementation Action Group) (n.d.). Speakers Notes on Seebohm. London: SIAG.

Simey, M. B. (1951). *Charitable Effort in Liverpool in the Nineteenth Century*. Liverpool: Liverpool Univeristy Press.

Simpkin, M. (1979). *Trapped within Welfare: Surviving Social Work*. London: Macmillan.

Sinfield, A. (1969). *Which Way for Social Work?* London: The Fabian Society.

Smith, L. and D. Jones (eds) (1981). *Deprivation, Participation and Community Action*. London: Routledge & Kegan Paul.

Social Work Reform Board (2011) Minutes of the Social Work Reform Board, www.education.gov.uk/swrb/b0074393/swrb-documents/minutes-of-the-social-work-reform-board (accessed 12 May 2011).

Social Work Task Force (2009). *Building a Safe, Confident Future*. London: Department for Children, Schools and Families.

Specht, H., Vickery, A. (1977). *Integrating Social Work Methods*. London: George Allen & Unwin.

Specht, H. and M. E. Courtney (1994). *Unfaithful Angels: How Social Work has Abandoned its Mission*. New York: The Free Press.

Spencer, H. (1884). *Man versus the State*. London: Williams & Norgate.

Starkey, P. (2000). 'The feckless mother: women, poverty and social workers in wartime and post-war England', *Women's History Review* **9**(3): 539–57.

Stears, M. (2001). *Progressives, Pluralists, and the Problems of the State: Ideologies of Reform in the United States and Britain 1909–1926*. Oxford: Oxford University Press.

Stedman Jones, G. (2004). *An End to Poverty? A Historical Debate*. London: Profile Books.

Stedman Jones, G. (1971). *Outcast London: A Study in the Relationship between Classes in Victorian Society*. Oxford: Clarendon Press.

Stein, M. (1997). *What Works in Leaving Care?* Ilford: Barnardo's Publications.

Stephens, T. (ed.) (1945). *Problem Families: An Experiment in Social Rehabilitation*. London: Pacifist Service Unit.

Stewart, J. (2006). 'Child guidance in interwar Scotland: international influences and domestic concerns', *Bulletin of the History of Medicine* **80**: 513–39.

Sturdy, H. and W. Parry-Jones (1999). 'Boarding-out insane patients: the significance of the Scottish system 1857–1913', in P. Bartlett and D. Wright (eds) *Outside the Walls of the Asylum: The History of Community Care 1750–2000*. London: The Athlone Press.

Sullivan, M. (2009). 'Social workers in community care practice: ideologies and interactions with older people', *British Journal of Social Work* **39**(7): 1306–25.

Szasz, T. S. (1960). 'The myth of mental illness', *American Psychologist* **15**: 113–18.

Taft, J. (1924). 'The use of the transfer within the limits of the office interview', *The Family* **5**(6): 145.

Taylor, L., R. Lacey and D. Bracken (1979). *In Whose Best Interests? The Unjust Treatment of Children in Courts and Institutions*. Nottingham: Cobden Trust and MIND.

Thomas, J. (1984). 'Bouquets and barbed wire', *Community Care*, January 5 Business Press International, p. 25.

Thomas, M. (2011). Personal communication.

Thomas, R. 'Fox, Dame Evelyn Emily Marian (1874–1955)', rev. *Oxford Dictionary of National Biography*. Oxford: Oxford University Press. Available at http://www.oxforddnb.com/view/article/33231 (accessed 7 July 2011).

Thompson, F. M. L. (ed.) (1990). *The Cambridge Social History of Britain 1750–1950*. Cambridge: Cambridge University Press.

Thomson, D. (1984). 'The decline of social welfare: falling state support for the elderly since early Victorian times', *Ageing and Society* **4**(4): 451–82.

Thomson, M. (2006). *Psychological Subjects: Identity, Culture, and Health in Twentieth Century Britain*. Oxford: Oxford University Press.

Thomson, M. (1998). *The Problem of Mental Deficiency: Eugenics, Democracy, and Social Policy in Britain c.1870–1959*. Oxford: Clarendon Press.

Timmins, N. (1995). *The Five Giants: A Biography of the Welfare State*. London: HarperCollins.

Timms, N. (1964). *Psychiatric Social Work in Great Britain 1939–1962*. London: Routledge.

Titmuss, R. (1968). *Commitment to Welfare*. London: Allen &Unwin.

Towle, C. (1941). *Social Case Records from Psychiatric Clinics*. Chicago: University of Chicago Press.

Townsend, D. (1984). 'Patrick Jenkin ought to know better …', *Community Care*, March 15 Business Press International, pp. 14–15.

Townshend, E. (1911). *The Case Against the Charity Organization Society*. London: The Fabian Society.

Tredgold, A. (1908). *Mental Deficiency*. London: Baillière Tindall & Cox.

Trevelyan, J. P. (1920). *Evening Play Centres for Children. The Story of their Origin and Growth*. London: Methuen.

Underwood, J. E. A. (1955). *Report of the Committee on Maladjusted Children* (Underwood Report). London: HMSO.

Utting, D., W. Rose and G. Pugh (2002). *Better Results for Children and Families: Involving Communities in Planning Services based on Outcomes*. London: NCVCCO.

Wagner, G. (1988). *Residential Care: A Positive Choice* (Wagner Report). London: National Institute for Social Work.

Walkowitz, D. (1999). *Working with Class: Social Workers and the Politics of Middle-Class Identity*. Chapel Hill: University of North Carolina Press.

Walkowitz, D. (1990). 'The making of a feminine professional identity: social workers in the 1920s', *American Historical Review* **95**(4): 1051–75.

Waterhouse, L. and J. McGhee (2002). 'Children's hearings in Scotland: compulsion and disadvantage', *Journal of Social Welfare and Family Law* **24**(3): 279–96.

Waterhouse, R. (2000). *Lost in Care: Report of the Tribunal of Inquiry into the Abuse of Children in Care*. London: The Stationery Office.

Waterson, J. (1999). 'Redefining community care social work: needs or risks led?' *Health and Social Care in the Community* **8**: 443–52.

Waugh, B. (1873). *The Gaol Cradle: Who Rocks It?* London: Strahan.

Webb, D. (1991). 'Puritans and paradigms: a speculation on the form of new moralities in social work', *Social Work and Social Sciences Review* **2**(2): 146–59.

Webb, J. (2011). Conversation with John Webb.

Webb, M. (2011). Conversation with Margot Webb.

Weiner, M. (1990). *Reconstructing the Criminal: Culture, Law and Policy in England 1830–1914*. Cambridge: Cambridge University Press.

Weinstein, J. (1984). 'Professionalism under pressure', *Community Care*, March 22 Business Press International, pp. 14–15.

Welshman, J. (1999). 'Rhetoric and reality: community care in England and Wales 1948–1974, in P. Bartlett and D. Wright (eds) *Outside the Walls of the Asylum: The History of Community Care 1750–2000*. London: The Athlone Press.

Westwood, L. (2007). 'Care in the community of the mentally disordered: the case of the Guardianship Society 1900–1939', *Social History of Medicine* **20**(1): 57–72.

Whelan, R. (2001). *Helping the Poor: Friendly Visiting, Dole-Charities and Dole Queues*. London: Civitas.

Whelan, R. (ed.) (1998). *Octavia Hill and the Social Housing Debate*, Rediscovered Riches series. London: IEA Health and Welfare Unit.

White, T. (2010). Conversation with Tom White.

White, T. (2011). *The Surprise of My Life*, privately published.

Wiener, M. (1996). *Reconstructing the Criminal: Culture, Law and Policy in England 1830–1914*. Cambridge: Cambridge University Press.

Willmott, P. (2004). 'London's School Care Committee Service 1908–1989', *Voluntary Action* **6**(2): 95–110.

Woodroofe, K. (1962). *From Charity to Social Work in England and the United States*. London: Routledge & Kegan Paul.

Woods, R. (1891). *English Social Movements*. New York: Scribner's Sons.

Wootton, B. (1959). *Social Science and Social Pathology*. London: George Allen & Unwin.

Yelling, J. A. (1999). *Slums and Redevelopment: Policy and Practice in England, 1918–45, with particular reference to London*. London: Taylor & Francis.

Yelling, J. A. (1986). *Slums and Slum Clearance in Victorian London*. London: Routledge.

Yelloly, M. (1980). *Social Work Theory and Psychoanalysis*. London: Van Nostrand Reinhold.

Young, A. F. and E. T. Ashton (1956). *British Social Work in the Nineteenth Century*. London: Routledge & Kegan Paul.

Younghusband, E. (1978). *Social Work in Britain, 1950–1975: A Follow-Up Study*. London: George Allen & Unwin.

Younghusband, E. (1947). *Report on the Employment and Training of Social Workers*. Carnegie United Kingdom Trust.

Younghusband Report (1959). *Report of the Committee on Social Workers in the Local Authority Health and Welfare Services*. London: HMSO.

Index

Addams, Jane 45
Adoption Act (1926) 98
Adoption Act (1949) 166–7
Adoption Act (1958) 166–7
Adoption of Children (Regulation) Act (1939) 98
Adrian, Hester 77
advocacy and self-advocacy movement 153–4
Agnew, E. 53
Ainsworth, Mary 164
Alden, Percy 45
Allen, Margery 164–5
Anglican strand in reform movement 9, 15–16
Anti-Slavery Society 9
approved social worker (ASW)
  discretionary powers of, problems with 202
  introduction of 202
  training and assessment of 202–3
Association of Child Care Officers (ACCO) 118, 119–20, 122, 166, 207
  legal basis for preventive work, pressure for 168–9
Association of Directors of Adult Social Services (ADASS) 200
Association of Family Caseworkers 122
Association of Hospital Almoners 60
Association of Moral Welfare Workers 122
Association of Psychiatric Social Workers 122
Association of Social Work (ASW) 122
Association of Social Workers 122
asylum system, expansion of 66–7
Atkinson, D., Jackson, M. and Walmsley, J. 65, 69, 79
Atlee, Clement 41, 51

Bailey, V. 99, 100
Bamford, T. 154, 197, 198

Barclay, Peter 141
Barclay Report (1982) 141–3, 206
  criticisms of 141
  influence of 142–3
Barnardo, Thomas John 91–2, 104n2
Barnett, Henrietta 36, 38
Barnett, Samuel 23, 36, 38, 39
Batty, D. 157
Beck, Frank 179–80
Beckford, Jasmine 175
Beers, Clifford 56
Behlmer, G.K. 92, 94–5, 95–6
Bell, E.M. 32–3, 59, 212
Bell, Steve 130, 134–5
Bell, Stuart 185n1
Bevan, Aneurin 165
Beveridge, William 41, 61, 62, 67
Beveridge Report (1942) 163
  publication of 108–9
Biestek, Father 112
'big society,' Social Work Reform Board and 161
Bilton, Keith 118, 208
Bion, Wilfred 112
Birmingham women's settlement 39–41
Bissell, V. 45
The Bitter Cry of Outcast London (Mearns, A.) 35
Booth, Charles 36
Bosanquet, Bernard 23, 29–30, 44, 53
Bosanquet, Helen 20–21, 23, 25, 30, 53, 57, 213
Boston Associated Charities, US 47
Bowlby, John 112, 113, 164
Bradley, Kate 48n2
Braye, S. 151
Braye, S. and Preston-Shoot, M. 151
Brewer, C. and Lait, J. 138
Brief and Extended Casework (Reid, W. and Shyne, A.W.) 115
Brill, K. and Thomas, R. 167

British Association of Social Workers
(BASW) 61, 206, 207–8
creation of 122–4
social workers strike, upheaval
within 138–9
British Federation of Social Workers
122
*Bulletin of the Association of Moral
Welfare Workers* 124
Burnett, R. and Appleton, C. 172
Burt, Cyril 57, 79, 100–101, 170
Butler-Sloss, L. 176, 177
Butterfield, Herbert 212

Cadbury, George 45
Cahill, M. and Jowitt, T. 47
Callaghan, Jim 117
Campbell, Beatrix 185n1
Caplan, Gerald 125
Care Council for Wales 156–7
care management 196–9
problems of 198
see also community care
Care Standards Act (2000) 156
Carer's Recognition and Services Act
(1995) 151
Carlisle, Kimberly 175
Case Con (radical social work journal)
128
manifesto 129–30
Case Conference (ASW journal) 122
casework
Brief and Extended Casework (Reid, W.
and Shyne, A.W.) 115
casework theory 111–12
consolidation between Wars of 52–4
Family Service Unit (FSU) definition
of 114
formalization of approaches
emergent from 125
individual uniqueness, fundamental
basis of 111
in mid-20th century 110–15
psychoanalysis and 112–14
social casework 110
systematization of 52–4
Wooton's critique of 114
writing on, COS and 24–5
Cashmore, Helen 42, 57
Cawthorn, Craig 112, 113, 136, 143,
152, 160, 166

Central Association for Mental Welfare
(CAMW) 68, 72, 73, 74, 75–6,
77, 80–81, 103
Central Council for Education and
Training in Social Work
(CCETSW) 145, 146, 147, 148,
154, 156, 202–3
Certificate of Qualification in Social
Work (CQSW) 154
Certificate of Social Service (CSS) 124,
154, 155
Chalmers, Thomas 12–15, 19
discussion point 13–14
individual attention, importance for
13
moral code within free market,
importance for 13
systematic house visiting scheme 12
visitor and visited, importance of
relationship between 13
Chamberlain, Joseph 39
*A Changing Psychology in Social Case
Work* (Robinson, V.) 56
Chaplin, Charlie 85–6
Charity Organisation Review (1876) 26–7
Charity Organisation Society (COS) 12,
16, 17, 18–34, 206, 211, 212,
213, 215
'character,' emphasis on 20–24
Chartist agitation for universal
suffrage 18
criticisms 29–31
decision-making procedures (and
outcomes) 27–8
defensive against imposition of state
aid 51–2
district committees, establishment of
19–20
economic circumstances, position of
society and 30–31
foundation and early decades 18–20
functions of, differing perspectives
on 33–4
further reading 34
Guilds of Help, Councils of Social
Service and 46, 47, 48
hospital almoners 31–3
idealism of founders 23–4
modernization efforts 31
moralizing tendencies and
ambivalence in thinking 21

origins of 19–20
outdoor relief, crusade against 19–20
poverty debate, position of society
	and 30–31
progressive political tide after 1900,
	antipathy towards 29
provincial societies, relief forms
	developed by 29
Reform Act (1867) 18
responsibility, emphasis on
	self-reliance and sense of 20
settlement house movement and 35,
	36, 38, 40, 42, 43, 44
social casework 24–9
social reform, position in history of
	33–4
state involvement in welfare
	provision, opposition to 29–30
summary 34
working-class behaviour, anxiety
	about 19
writing on casework 24–5
Chartists, agitation for universal
	suffrage 18
Child Care Act (1980) 179
Child Guidance Council (1927) 60
Children Act (1889) 93–4
Children Act (1908) 95–6, 102
Children Act (1933) 165
Children Act (1948) 165–6, 167
Children Act (1975) 136
Children Act (1989) 151, 181–3
Children Act (2004) 183–4
Children and Young Persons Act
	(1933) 102
Children and Young Persons Act
	(1963) 169, 170
Children and Young Persons Act
	(1969) 136, 170–71, 179
Children Who Wait (Rowe, J. and
	Lambert, L.) 178
Christian socialism 22, 38
Chronically Sick and Disabled Act
	(1970) 136, 151, 193
Church of England Temperance
	Society 99–100, 103, 206
Clarke, J. 192
Clement Brown, S. 56
Cleveland, crisis in 176–7
Butler-Sloss recommendations 177
Climbié, Victoria 183

Clyde Report (1946) 165
College of Social Work 208
Colwell, Maria 174–5, 185
commissioning, competences and
	'social care' 148–62
advocacy and self-advocacy
	movement 153–4
'big society,' Social Work Reform
	Board and 161
Care Council for Wales 156–7
care services, difficulties of
	judgements about provision
	149
Care Standards Act (2000) 156
Certificate of Qualification in Social
	Work (CQSW) 154
choice, difficulties of 151–3
contract culture, state involvement
	in 149
DipSW 154, 155
further reading 162
General Social Care Council (GSCC)
	156–8, 161
individual control and
	personalization, steps towards
	151
market and welfare state, conflict
	between objectives of 148–9
MIND 60, 110, 153, 193, 194, 202
National Vocational Qualification
	(NVQ) 157–8
New Public Management (NPM)
	150–51
NHS and Community Care Act
	(1990) 149, 156
Northern Ireland Social Care Council
	156–7
office-based social work 150–51
professional qualifications, reform of
	154–8
qualifying training, question of
	154–5
SANE 153
Scottish Social Services Council
	156–7
service users, gains in influence for
	151–4
social work
	coalition government attitudes
	towards 161
	'core,' size of 160

commissioning, competences and
'social care' (*Continued*)
marketplace and 148–51
procedures, exercise of
independent judgement and
155–6
Social Work Reform Board 160, 161
Social Work Task Force (SWTF)
158–60, 161
definition of social work 159–60
recommendations of 159
social work tasks, user groups and
definition of 158
summary 161–2
Training Organization for Personal
Social Services (TOPSS) 157
transition to post-Seebohm
departments, negativity in 150
Union of the Physically Impaired
Against Segregation (UPIAS)
152–3
Commonwealth Fund 61
community care 66, 70, 79–80, 149,
186, 197, 198
failures of 193
mental disorder and first phase of
187–94
older people and second phase of
194–6
personalization and third phase of
199–201
social worker supply and 191
see also care management
Community Care 124, 138, 139, 150,
202, 203
Community Care (Direct Payments)
Act (1996) 151
community social work 140–41
Congregationalist strand in reform
movement 15–16
Connor, Herbert 76, 77–8
Conservative Party 51, 100, 108, 132,
209–10
in government 18, 120, 129, 138,
141, 145–6, 148, 154, 157, 191
contract culture, state involvement in
149
Cooper, J. 115, 116
Corby, B. 175
Corrigan, P. 144
Corrigan, P. and Leonard, P. 129

Councils of Social Service 46–8
Councils of Social Welfare 46, 47,
51–2, 82
Cretney, Stephen 167
Crime: A Challenge to Us All (Longford,
G.A.) 116
Criminal Justice Act (1925) 100
Crippled Children's Union 40
The Crisis of Liberalism (Hobson, J.)
48n3
Crosland, Anthony 127–8
Crossman, Richard 117
Cullen, L. 31
Cummins, Anne 32–3
Curtis, Myra 165
Curtis Report (1946) 165, 167

Darwin, Charles 68
Darwinism 24
social Darwinism 67–8
Davies, Martin 144, 196
Dendy, Mary 68–9, 71–2, 76
Denison, Edward 36
Depression 61–3
Digby, A. 67
DipSW 154, 155, 206
Disabled Persons (Services,
Consultation and
Representation) Act (1986) 151
discussion points
assessments and referrals, decisions
about 149
care management changes, turning
back the clock? 153
Case Con manifesto 130
Charity Organization Society
casework and decision-making
26–7
child abuse, reactions to pressures on
178
community social work 143
long-term fostering, decisions about
179
Marxism of maintenance? 144
mental deficiencies, attitudes
towards those with 69
Mental Deficiency Act (1913) 71
Octavia Hill, for or against 21–3
Pindown regime, what were they
thinking? 181
settlement house principles 42

Newcastle Board of Guardians 37
NHS and Community Care Act (1990)
    149, 156, 196–9, 208
  consequences of 198–9
Northern Ireland Social Care Council
    156–7
Norwood Orphanage 90
Nussey, Helen 59

Oliver, Michael 153
O'Neill, Dennis 164
On the Origin of Species (Darwin, C.) 68
Orme, J. 154, 155, 157, 158
Our Health, Our Care, Our Say (DoH,
    2006) 151
Oxford Dictionary of National Biography
    213

Packman, J. 167, 168, 169, 170
Pankhurst, Emmeline 37, 88–9
Parton, N. 174
Payne, M. 124, 201–2
Penketh, L. 145–6
People's Free Kindergarten Association
    41
Perlman, Helen 112
Philpot, Terry 91, 117, 124, 139, 170
Pierson, J. 146
'Pindown' regime 180–81
Pinker, Robert 142–3, 146, 209
Pinsent, Ellen 76–7
Pollitt, C. 210
Poor Law (1601), welfare system of 7–8
Poor Law Amendment Act (1834) 7–9
  children under 85–90
  deterrence of applications for poor
    relief 8, 9
  dismantlement of 62–3
  eligibility for poor relief under 8
  outdoor relies, tradition in Scotland
    of 9
  Poor Law Board 16
  Poor Law Commission 8, 16
  poor law principles, introduction to
    Ireland of 9
  Poor Law Unions 8, 9, 16–17
  poor relief based on 8
  Royal Commission into the
    Operation of the Poor Laws 8
  summary 17
  workhouse building 9, 15

Poor Man's Lawyer Association 41
Postle, Karen 152
practical socialism 38
Pringle, J. 55
Prior, P. 202
Prison Discipline Society 9
Prochaska, F. 22
professional qualifications, reform of
    154–8
Progress: Civic, Social and Industrial 45
psychiatric social workers (PSWs)
  elitist aspirations 60–61
  emergence of 57
  social work with adults 189–90
Purcell, Anne 95–6
Putting People First (DoH, 2007) 200,
    201
Puxley, Zoe 97–8

Quaker strand in reform movement 9
Quality Strategy for Social Care (DoH,
    2000) 155

radical social work
  emergence of 128–30
  legacy of 140–43
  rationale for emergence in 1970s
    128–30
radical voices, turbulent times 127–47
  anti-capitalism 129
  anti-racism and anti-oppressive
    practice 145–6
  Barclay Report (1982), influence of
    141–3
  Case Con manifesto 129–30
  Community Care, voice and advocacy
    of 139
  community social work 140–41
  conflict within social work,
    professionalization or
    unionization 131–6
  economic crisis (1976), effects of
    127–8
  further reading 147
  institutional racism, Macpherson
    definition of 146
  National Association of Local
    Government Officers (NALGO)
    131, 136–8
  National Union of Public Employees
    (NUPE) 131, 132–3, 134, 136–7

radical voices, turbulent times
(*Continued*)
social capital 142
social work, trade union or
profession? 130–36
social work as maintenance 143–5
social workers
class origins of 129
strike of 136–9
strike by social workers
demands of unions 136–7
long-tern effects 138
settlement agreement 137
union case for 136
summary 146–7
trade union decline 138
trade union influence 131
trade union membership 131
welfare state
origins of 130
social work within 133–6
Rathbone, Elizabeth 98, 109
Reform Act (1867) 18
Reid, W. and Epstein, L. 115, 125
Reid, W. and Shyne, A.W. 115
Ricardo, David 6, 10
Richmond, Mary 25, 46–7, 50, 52–4,
59–60, 63, 111, 114
Rimmer, J. 39–41, 42, 43
Roberts, M.J.D. 15
Robinson, Sarah and Alfred 86
Robinson, Virginia 56
Rodgers, D. 45, 46
Rogowski, S. 150
Rolph, S., Atkinson, D. and Walmsley,
J. 187–9, 192
Rooff, M. 68, 212
Rose, Nikolas 216
Rowe, J. and Lambert, L. 178
Rowntree, Seebohm 36, 45, 50, 62
Royal Commission into the Operation
of the Poor Laws 8
Royal Commission on Mental Health
190–91
Royal Commission on the Care and
Control of the Feeble-Minded
68, 69
Royal Commission on the Poor Laws
and Relief of Distress 213
Royal Society for the Prevention of
Cruelty to Animals (RSPCA) 93

Roycroft, Brian 136
Rummery, K. and Glendinning, C. 152,
194
Ruskin, John 19, 22

Sainsbury, Eric 115
Salem Comes to the Boro (Bell, S.) 185n1
Sandlebridge Colony, Cheshire 71–2
Satyamurti, C. 121–2, 136
Sayce, L. 194
Scarman Report (1982) 145
Schafer, A. 45
Schön, D.A. 125
Scottish Social Services Council 156–7
Seebohm, Frederic 117
Seebohm Committee
Report (1968) 117–18, 119, 121
and single social services department
107, 115–20
Seebohm Implementation Action
Group (SIAG) 118–19
Seed, P. 212
settlement house movement 35–44,
48–9
activities and services, range of 40–41
adult education, involvement in 44
Birmingham women's settlement
39–41
contribution to social work 41–2
democratization (limited) of relief 36
early social work training and 42–3
expansion of 39–41
fellowship, sense of 38
further reading 49
medical care 40–41
neighbourhoods, holistic approach
to 38–9
origins of 36–41
poverty and destitution in London
36
provident society savings scheme 40
residency, notion of 38
resident settlers, objectives for 39
Scottish settlements and social work
training 44
summary 48
Toynbee Hall 36, 38, 39, 41, 45–6,
48n2
workhouse system 35–6
Sewell, Margaret 42, 43, 57
Simey, Margaret B. 10, 11–12, 57–8

social work history, assessment of interpretations of 216
Social Work Task Force, definition of social work 160
Thomas Chalmers, legacy of 13–14
working with the 'mentally defective' 78
Disinherited Youth (Carnegie Trust) 62
Disraeli, Benjamin 18
Domestic Mission Report (1837) 11–12
Dominelli, L. 150
Donnison, D., Jay, P. and Stewart, M. 115–16
Dr Barnardo's 90, 91–2
duly authorized officers (DAOs) 187–9
Dumsday, W. and Moss, J. 66
Dunleavy, P. and Hood, C. 150

Eaton, L. 193
Ehrenreich, J.H. 215
Elberfeld district visiting system 47
Elementary Education (Defective and Epileptic Children) Act (1899) 71
Ellis, K., Davis, A. and Rummery, K. 121
Etzioni, A. 58
eugenics 213
   eugenics movement 68
evangelism and social work 9–10
Evening Argus (Brighton) 174
Every Child Matters (2003) 183–4

Factory Acts (1833 and 1844) 7
Fair Access to Care Services (FACS, DoH, 2003) 199
Family Service Unit (FSU) 114
Father Hudson Society 90
Finkelstein, V. 152
Finlayson, G. 46, 62, 67
First World War 50–51
Fisher, T. 174
Flexner, Abraham 60, 207
Folbre, Nancy 211
Forward 47
Foucault, Michel 215
Fox, Evelyn 74, 213
Frere, M. 89–90
Freud, Anna 112
Freud, Sigmund 55, 112, 113
Friedson, E. 207

Fry, Margery 99–100
Furgol, M.T. 14
further reading
   Charity Organisation Society (COS) 34
   commissioning, competences and 'social care' 162
   'mental deficiency,' working with 83
   radical voices, turbulent times 147
   settlement house movement 49
   social work between the Wars 64
   social work forerunners 17
   social work high tide 126
   social work with adults 204
   social work with children and young people 185
   welfare of children 104

Gabriel, J.M. 56
Geddes, Patrick 46
General Social Care Council (GSCC) 156–8, 161, 211
generic service department
   agreement on 117–18
   idea of 116–17
   pressures on 121–2
   shaping of 120–22
   'single door' premise of 121
Gladstone, William Ewart 19
Glover-Thomas, N. 70
Glueck, B. 57
Goffman, Erving 193
Goldstein, J., Freud, A. and Solnit, A. 171–2
Goodlad, L. 12, 13
Goschen, J.G. 19
Gostin, Larry 202
Green, T.H. 23–4
Griffiths Report (1988) 151, 161
Guardian 130
guardians, boards of 8, 16, 19, 70, 81
   Jewish Board of Guardians 59
   local boards, establishment of 36
   Newcastle Board of Guardians 37
   relieving officers (ROs), independence from 66
   transfer of functions to public assistance committees 62
   Wakefield Board of Guardians 69
Guardianship Act (1925) 98

Guilds of Help 46–8
  Councils of Social Service and 46, 47, 48
  district visiting system 47
  launch in Bradford of first Guild 46–7
  summary 48

Hadley, Roger 142–3
Hall, William Clarke 99–100, 117–18, 170
Hancock Nunn, Thomas 47
Handler, J. 169
Hanvey, C. 208
Hardie, Keir 46
Hardiker, P. and Barker, M. 125
Harris, John 150
Harris, Jose 23
Harrison, B. 48n3
Health and Social Care Act (2001) 151
Healy, William 57
Henry, Tyra 175
Heywood, J. 87, 88, 166
Hill, M. 121
Hill, Octavia 21–3, 25, 38, 42–3, 57, 212
Hilton, B. 13
Hilton, Boyd 212
Hobsbawm, E. 8
Hobson, J.A. 45
Holman, Bob 108, 163–4, 167
Homes of the London Poor (Hill, O.) 23
Hoppen, T. 19
Horsburgh, Florence 98
Hospital Almoners Association 60
Howard League for Penal Reform 99–100
Humphreys, R. 16–17, 20, 27, 29
Hunnybun, N. 190

Illich, Ivan 131
Independent Labour Party (ILP) 46, 47
industrial revolution 5–7
  Factory Acts (1833 and 1844) 7
  laissez-faire economics 6–7, 10
    power of 6–7
  market forces, dominance of 6
  mass migration, rural to urban 5
  mechanization 5
  mine and mill ownership 7
  moral revolution and 9

  political economy, 'dismal science' of 6
  poverty generation, epic scale of 8
  social problems of industrialization 5–6
  social work, origins in 9–15
  summary 17
  urban manufacturing centres 7
  urban population growth 5–6
Ingleby Committee (1960) 169, 172
Institute of Medical Social Workers 122
Institute of Psychiatric Social Workers 207
institutional abuse 179–80
institutional racism, Macpherson definition of 146
Inter-departmental Committee on Physical Deterioration 67

Jackson, M. 71–2
Jackson, S. 178
Jarrett, Mary C. 56, 64n2
Jennings, H. 89, 90
Jewish Board of Guardians 59
JM Consulting 154
Johns, Reverend John 11
Johnson, Liam 175
Jones, C. 150
Jordan, B. 152
Joseph, Keith 120

Kahan, Barbara 169–70
Keating, J. 87, 96, 97
Kellogg, P. and Gleason, A. 46
Kellogg, Paul 46
Kempe, Henry 173–4, 176
Kemshall, H. et al. 149
Kendall, K.A. 43
Kenworthy, Marion 56, 57
Kilbrandon Committee (and Report) in (1960-64) Scotland 172–3
Klein, Melanie 112
Koseda, Heidi 175

Labour and the New Social Order (1918) 50
Labour Party 29, 41, 46, 50–51, 52, 108–9
Lady Derby's Benevolent Society 10
laissez-faire economics 6–7, 10
Laming, Lord 183

Leadbetter, C. 200
Lee, Porter 56, 57
Leighton, B. 36
Leonard, Peter 135–6, 144, 214
Letters (Hill, O.) 23
Levy, A. and Kahan, B. 181
Lewis, J. 21, 30, 47, 51, 52
Liberal Party 19, 23, 30, 37, 39, 212
   in government 29, 30, 45
Lindemann, Erich 125
Lindsay, Mike 153
Liverpool District Provident Society 10
Lloyd, L. 152
Local Authority Social Services Act
   (1970) 119–20
Local Government Act (1929) 62, 63,
   101–2
Local Government Board 16–17
Loch, Charles Stewart 25, 30, 31, 38,
   44, 52–3
London Association for the Care of the
   Mentally Defective 76
London County Council (LCC) 57, 62,
   75, 76, 80, 89, 100
London School of Economics (LSE) 61
Longford, Lord 116
Lost in Care (Millham, S., Bullock, R.
   et al.) 178
Lowe, G.R. and Reid, P.N. 214–15
Lowe, R. 50
Lubove, R. 53, 215
Lunacy Act (1890) 67
Lunacy Commission 66
Lunacy (Scotland) Act (1857) 66
Lunbeck, E. 56
Lymbery, M. 149

Macadam, Elizabeth 51, 62, 63
MacDonald, Ramsey 46
McDougall, K. and Cormack, U.
   109–10, 110–11
McGoldrick, Karl 175
MacPherson Report (1999) 146
Manthorpe, J. 43
Margolin, Leslie 33, 215
Marshall, Mary 195–6, 209
Matrimonial Causes Act (1857) 85
Meacham, S. 24, 38, 39
Mearns, Arthur 35
Medical Social Work 124
Men Without Work (Pilgrim Trust) 62

Mendicity Society 15
Mental After Care Association 75–6
Mental Capacity Act (2005) 201
'mental deficiency,' working with
   65–83
   asylum system, expansion of 66–7
   child guidance, partnership model
      on 81
   citizenship, question of 80
   colonies, growth of 73
   colony model, development of 72–3
   eugenics movement 68
   further reading 83
   guardians *in loco parentis* 70
   guardianship 79
   institutionalization 66
   labour market, protections from
      rigours of 68–9
   learning disabilities
      case study of supervision
         (1919–34) of person with 77–8
      hereditary transmission of 67–8
      services for those with 68–9
   legal responsibility for ascertained
      defectives 79–80
   London, advanced nature of social
      work practice in 76
   lunacy and mental deficiency under
      Poor Law 65–7
   lunatic, 1845 definition 66
   Mental Deficiency Act (1913) 70–72
      campaign for 69, 72
   Mental Deficiency (Amendment) Act
      (1927) 80
   Mental Deficiency and Lunacy Act
      (1913) 66, 68
   national fitness, social Darwinism
      and 67–8
   operation of 1913 Act, example of
      77–8
   physical deterioration, concerns
      about 67
   progressive ethos, first steps towards
      80–81
   psychotherapy, partnership model
      on 81
   relieving officers 66–7
   segregation 72–3
   service in the community, expansion
      of 79–82
   sexualized behaviour 78–9

'mental deficiency,' working with
(*Continued*)
social Darwinism 67–8
social work services, decision-making
procedures, fragmentary nature
of 75–6
social work tasks under 1913 Act,
fragmentation and dispersal of
74–5
social workers and mental deficiency
73–8
summary 82
supervision 75–8, 79–80
supervisory role, contradictions in 75
surveillance and control systems,
establishment of 70
terminological change (1960s) 81
terminology of earlier times,
crudeness of 65
visiting committees 66–7
voluntary hostels, establishment of
73
women and mental deficiency 78–9
Mental Deficiency Act (1913) 60, 70–72
campaign for 69, 72
Mental Deficiency (Amendment) Act
(1927) 80
Mental Deficiency and Lunacy Act
(1913) 66, 68
Mental Health Act (1959) 70, 188, 191,
203
Mental Health Act (1983) 202
Mental Hygiene and Social Work (Lee, P.
and Kenworthy, M.) 56
Mental Welfare Association 192
Mental Welfare News 124
Mental Welfare Officers Society 187
Methodist strand in reform movement
9, 15–16
Metropolitan Visiting and Relief
Association 16
Meyer, Adolf 57
Miller, Harry 44
Millham, S., Bullock, R. et al. 178
MIND 60, 110, 153, 193, 202
campaign objectives 194
A Mind that Found Itself (Beers, C.) 56
Monckton Report (1945) 164
Moore, M.J. 46, 47
Moorehouse, M. 69
Morris, C. 56

Munro, E. and Calder, M. 184
Murphy, J. 173
The Myth of Mental Illness (Szasz, T.) 192

National Adoption Society (NAS) 97
National Assistance Act (1948) 186,
193, 201
National Association for the Welfare of
the Feeble-Minded 68, 69
National Association of Local
Government Officers (NALGO)
131, 136–8
National Association of Mental Health
60
formation of 110
National Association of Probation
Officers 122
National Association of Social Workers
(US) 215–16
National Children Adoption
Association (NCAA) 97
National Children's Homes 90, 91
National Council for Mental Hygiene
(1922) 60
national fitness, social Darwinism and
67–8
National Health Service Act (1946) 186
National Institute for Social Work
(NISW) 116, 117, 141, 194–5
National Liberals 108
National Society for the Prevention of
Cruelty to Children (NSPCC)
206, 210–11
child abuse
and child protection (1970s and
1980s) 174
definition of 93
cruelty to children, cases of 94
professionalism of inspectorate 94–5
records (1898), extract from 95–6
role of 'cruelty man' within
working-class families 94–5
welfare of children 92–6
National Union of Public Employees
(NUPE) 131, 132–3, 134, 136–7
National Union of Women Workers
39–40
National Vocational Qualification
(NVQ) 157–8
New Public Management (NPM)
150–51

Newcastle Board of Guardians 37
NHS and Community Care Act (1990)
    149, 156, 196–9, 208
  consequences of 198–9
Northern Ireland Social Care Council
    156–7
Norwood Orphanage 90
Nussey, Helen 59

Oliver, Michael 153
O'Neill, Dennis 164
On the Origin of Species (Darwin, C.) 68
Orme, J. 154, 155, 157, 158
Our Health, Our Care, Our Say (DoH,
    2006) 151
Oxford Dictionary of National Biography
    213

Packman, J. 167, 168, 169, 170
Pankhurst, Emmeline 37, 88–9
Parton, N. 174
Payne, M. 124, 201–2
Penketh, L. 145–6
People's Free Kindergarten Association
    41
Perlman, Helen 112
Philpot, Terry 91, 117, 124, 139, 170
Pierson, J. 146
'Pindown' regime 180–81
Pinker, Robert 142–3, 146, 209
Pinsent, Ellen 76–7
Pollitt, C. 210
Poor Law (1601), welfare system of 7–8
Poor Law Amendment Act (1834) 7–9
  children under 85–90
  deterrence of applications for poor
    relief 8, 9
  dismantlement of 62–3
  eligibility for poor relief under 8
  outdoor relies, tradition in Scotland
    of 9
  Poor Law Board 16
  Poor Law Commission 8, 16
  poor law principles, introduction to
    Ireland of 9
  Poor Law Unions 8, 9, 16–17
  poor relief based on 8
  Royal Commission into the
    Operation of the Poor Laws 8
  summary 17
  workhouse building 9, 15

Poor Man's Lawyer Association 41
Postle, Karen 152
practical socialism 38
Pringle, J. 55
Prior, P. 202
Prison Discipline Society 9
Prochaska, F. 22
professional qualifications, reform of
    154–8
Progress: Civic, Social and Industrial 45
psychiatric social workers (PSWs)
  elitist aspirations 60–61
  emergence of 57
  social work with adults 189–90
Purcell, Anne 95–6
Putting People First (DoH, 2007) 200,
    201
Puxley, Zoe 97–8

Quaker strand in reform movement 9
Quality Strategy for Social Care (DoH,
    2000) 155

radical social work
  emergence of 128–30
  legacy of 140–43
  rationale for emergence in 1970s
    128–30
radical voices, turbulent times 127–47
  anti-capitalism 129
  anti-racism and anti-oppressive
    practice 145–6
  Barclay Report (1982), influence of
    141–3
  Case Con manifesto 129–30
  Community Care, voice and advocacy
    of 139
  community social work 140–41
  conflict within social work,
    professionalization or
    unionization 131–6
  economic crisis (1976), effects of
    127–8
  further reading 147
  institutional racism, Macpherson
    definition of 146
  National Association of Local
    Government Officers (NALGO)
    131, 136–8
  National Union of Public Employees
    (NUPE) 131, 132–3, 134, 136–7

radical voices, turbulent times
(*Continued*)
social capital 142
social work, trade union or
profession? 130–36
social work as maintenance 143–5
social workers
class origins of 129
strike of 136–9
strike by social workers
demands of unions 136–7
long-tern effects 138
settlement agreement 137
union case for 136
summary 146–7
trade union decline 138
trade union influence 131
trade union membership 131
welfare state
origins of 130
social work within 133–6
Rathbone, Elizabeth 98, 109
Reform Act (1867) 18
Reid, W. and Epstein, L. 115, 125
Reid, W. and Shyne, A.W. 115
Ricardo, David 6, 10
Richmond, Mary 25, 46–7, 50, 52–4,
59–60, 63, 111, 114
Rimmer, J. 39–41, 42, 43
Roberts, M.J.D. 15
Robinson, Sarah and Alfred 86
Robinson, Virginia 56
Rodgers, D. 45, 46
Rogowski, S. 150
Rolph, S., Atkinson, D. and Walmsley,
J. 187–9, 192
Rooff, M. 68, 212
Rose, Nikolas 216
Rowe, J. and Lambert, L. 178
Rowntree, Seebohm 36, 45, 50, 62
Royal Commission into the Operation
of the Poor Laws 8
Royal Commission on Mental Health
190–91
Royal Commission on the Care and
Control of the Feeble-Minded
68, 69
Royal Commission on the Poor Laws
and Relief of Distress 213
Royal Society for the Prevention of
Cruelty to Animals (RSPCA) 93

Roycroft, Brian 136
Rummery, K. and Glendinning, C. 152,
194
Ruskin, John 19, 22

Sainsbury, Eric 115
Salem Comes to the Boro (Bell, S.) 185n1
Sandlebridge Colony, Cheshire 71–2
Satyamurti, C. 121–2, 136
Sayce, L. 194
Scarman Report (1982) 145
Schafer, A. 45
Schön, D.A. 125
Scottish Social Services Council 156–7
Seebohm, Frederic 117
Seebohm Committee
Report (1968) 117–18, 119, 121
and single social services department
107, 115–20
Seebohm Implementation Action
Group (SIAG) 118–19
Seed, P. 212
settlement house movement 35–44,
48–9
activities and services, range of 40–41
adult education, involvement in 44
Birmingham women's settlement
39–41
contribution to social work 41–2
democratization (limited) of relief 36
early social work training and 42–3
expansion of 39–41
fellowship, sense of 38
further reading 49
medical care 40–41
neighbourhoods, holistic approach
to 38–9
origins of 36–41
poverty and destitution in London
36
provident society savings scheme 40
residency, notion of 38
resident settlers, objectives for 39
Scottish settlements and social work
training 44
summary 48
Toynbee Hall 36, 38, 39, 41, 45–6,
48n2
workhouse system 35–6
Sewell, Margaret 42, 43, 57
Simey, Margaret B. 10, 11–12, 57–8

Sisyphus 209
social capital 142
social casework 110
  social work methods and 115
social control
  notion of 216
  social work and 215–16
social Darwinism 67–8
Social Diagnosis (Richmond, M.) 53,
  60
social work
  attitude towards poor, hardening of
    11
  charitable activity, voluntary
    associations and 15–17
  Charity Organisation Society 12, 16,
    17
  children's services on eve of Second
    World War 103
  coalition government attitudes
    towards 161
  conflict within, professionalization
    or unionization 131–6
  'core,' size of 160
  District Provident Society in
    Liverpool 10
  Domestic Mission Report (1837)
    11–12
  as ensemble of functions 206–7
  evangelism and 9–10
  forerunners of 9–15
  functions, emergence of 88–90
  Lady Derby's Benevolent Society 10
  Local Government Board 16–17
  as maintenance 143–5
  marketplace and 148–51
  Mendicity Society 15
  method, unification of 124–5
  Metropolitan Visiting and Relief
    Association 16
  organisation, culture of 210
  origins in industrial revolution 9–15
  outdoor relief in London, growth of
    16
  perspectives before First World War,
    plurality of 45–8
  political economy, dominance of
    14–15
  poverty, moral condition of 11
  procedures, exercise of independent
    judgement and 155–6

  psychoanalysis and 112–13
  reform movement and 9–10
  responsible behaviour, promotion of
    11
  sectarian antagonisms, problem of
    16
  services for adults on eve of Second
    World War 82
  social work teams 121–2
  tasks under 1913 Act, fragmentation
    and dispersal of 74–5
  timeline (1819-1939) 2–3
  timeline (1939-2010) 106
  trade union or profession? 130–36
  voluntary associations and charitable
    activity 15–17
social work, high tide for
  Association of Child Care Officers
    (ACCO) 118, 119–20, 122
  Beveridge Report (1942), publication
    of 108–9
  British Association of Social Workers
    (BASW), creation of 122–4
  casework, Family Service Unit (FSU)
    definition of 114
  casework in mid-20th century
    110–15
  casework theory 111–12
  family department, notion of 116
  Family Service Unit (FSU) 114
  formalization of approaches
    emergent from casework 125
  further reading 126
  generic service department
    agreement on 117–18
    idea of 116–17
    pressures on 121–2
    shaping of 120–22
    'single door' premise of 121
  home front organization, wartime
    need for 108
  individual uniqueness, fundamental
    basis of casework 111
  Local Authority Social Services Act
    (1970) 119–20
  National Association of Mental
    Health, formation of 110
  National Institute for Social Work
    (NISW) 116, 117, 141, 194–5
  psychoanalysis, casework and
    112–14

social work, high tide for (*Continued*)
  Seebohm Committee and single
    social services department 107,
    115–20
  Seebohm Committee Report (1968)
    117–19
  Seebohm Implementation Action
    Group (SIAG) 118–19
  social casework 110
    social work methods and 115
  social compact between state and
    citizen (1946-1959) 109–1–
  social histories 111
  social work and psychoanalysis
    112–13
  social work method, unification of
    124–5
  social work teams 121–2
  Standing Conference of
    Organizations of Social Workers
    118
  summary 125
  wartime evacuation of children 108
  welfare state 107–9
    key legislation of 109
  Wooton's critique of casework 114
social work between the Wars 50–64
  autonomy of women in social work
    environments 58–9
  casework, consolidation of 52–4
  dependency, reappraisal of causes of
    53–4
  Depression 61–3
  early professional associations 60, 61
  family relationships, social systems
    theory and 53–4
  First World War, changes in attitudes
    after 50–52
  further reading 64
  local social service organizations,
    advocacy for 63
  mental hygiene 56–7
  political landscape, rightward
    movement of 51
  Poor Law, dismantlement of 62–3
  professional status, quest for 57–61
  psychiatric social worker
    elitist aspirations 60–61
    emergence of 57
  psychological knowledge, case work
    redesign in light of 55–6

  'psychological turn' 54–6
  public sector, post First World War
    attitudes 51–2
  social problem families, references to
    55
  summary 63–4
  systematization of casework 52–4
  terminology, changes in 55, 56
  United States, comparison with 55
  Victorian notions of respectability,
    challenges to 58
  voluntary expertise, local
    government incorporation of 63
  voluntary organizations,
    collaboration with local
    authorities 51–2
  voluntary sector, post First World
    War attitudes 51–2
  women and professional status 58
  women's professional aspirations,
    scope for 57–60
social work history 211
  adaptive nature of social work 206–7
  College of Social Work 208
  compassionate conservatism 212–13
  conclusive solutions, lack of 210
  corporate management techniques,
    introduction of 214
  defining social work 205–7
  eugenics 213
  exclusion, tackling roots of 209–10
  function, sought or imposed,
    expansion of 206
  gender considerations 210–11
  gender imbalance 211
  global economic crisis (2008-9),
    insoluble contradictions
    produced by 214
  interpretation of 211–16
  labour costs, problem of 209
  market and public sector, argument
    over rival virtues 208–9
  Marxist interpretations 213–14
  multifaceted nature of social work
    206–7
  pendulum phenomenon 210
  pink collar penalties 211
  professional recognition, aim of 215
  professional self-advancement,
    narrative of 214–15
  professional status, quest for 207–8

professionalisation of poverty
214–15
public and private services, boundary
between? 208–9
recognition as 'profession' 207
recurring themes in 205–11
social control
notion of 216
social work and 215–16
social democracy 208–9
social exclusion and social work
209–10
social work as ensemble of functions
206–7
social work organisation, culture of
210
welfare state, working-class efforts
towards 214
'Whig' interpretations 212–13
Social Work Reform Board 160, 161
Social Work (Scotland) Act (1968)
120
Social Work Task Force (SWTF) 206
commissioning, competences and
'social care' 158–60, 161
definition of social work 159–60
recommendations of 159
Social Work Today 124, 202
social work with adults 186–204
anti-psychiatry movement 192–3
approved social worker (ASW)
discretionary powers of, problems
with 202
introduction of 202
training and assessment of 202–3
care management 196–9
problems of 198
community care
failures of 193
social worker supply and 191
deprivation of liberty, safeguarding
and 201–3
division of labour, NHS and 187
duly authorized officers (DAOs)
187–9
eligibility criteria, *Fair Access to Care
Services* (FACS) and 199
further reading 204
Mental Capacity Act (2005) 201
mental disorder, community care
(first phase) and 187–94

Mental Health Act (1959) 188, 191,
203
Mental Health Act (1983) 202
mental health problems,
collaborative approaches to 189
Mental Welfare Association 192
mental welfare officers 191–2
Mental Welfare Officers Society 187
NHS and Community Care Act
(1990) 196–9
consequences of 198–9
older people, community care
(second phase) and 194–6
personalization
community care (third phase) and
199–201
principle of 199–201
postwar work with adults 186–7
psychiatric beds, fall in numbers
available 201
psychiatric social workers (PSWs)
189–90
purchaser-provider split, internal
market and 197–8
Royal Commission on Mental Health
190–91
social work and reform 190–94
subnormality, language of 189
summary 203
violence committed by adults under
supervision 201–2
Wagner Committee (and Report,
1987) 195
social work with children and young
people 163–85
Adoption Act (1949) 166–7
Adoption Act (1958) 166–7
Association of Child Care Officers
(ACCO) 166
legal bases for preventive work,
pressure for 168–9
'boarding out' officers 167
care or supervision orders, grounds
for 171–2
child abuse and protection (1970s
and 1980s) 173–8
Child Care Act (1980) 179
Children Act (1933) 165
Children Act (1948) 165–6, 167
Children Act (1989) 181–3
Children Act (2004) 183–4

social work with children and young
people (*Continued*)
Children and Young Persons Act
(1963) 169, 170
Children and Young Persons Act
(1969) 170–71, 179
children's departments, ethos and
practice 166–7
children's homes, 'humanization' of
167
Cleveland, crisis in 176–7
Butler-Sloss recommendations 177
Clyde Report (1946) 165
compulsory removal from families,
conflict over 167
cooperation, partnership working
and 170
corporate parent, local authority as
178–81
Curtis Report (1946) 165
Dennis O'Neill, death of 164
developments leading to Children
Act (1948) 164–6
Every Child Matters (2003) 183–4
experiences of children separated
from parents 164
further reading 185
government responses to young
offending, vacillation of 172
homelessness 168
Ingleby Committee (and Report) in
England 169, 172
institutional abuse 179–80
Kilbrandon Committee (and Report)
in Scotland 172–3
local authority as corporate parent
178–81
Maria Colwell, death of 174–5
most difficult years (mid-1980s)
175–6
permanency planning 179
'Pindown' regime 180–81
preventative work, development of
case for 167–70
public opinion, reconstruction of
children's services and 164–5
restoration to natural home when
appropriate, requirement for
165–6
Scotland, children's hearings in
172–3

separation, emotional needs and
163–4
social enquiry reports 171
social work expertise, legal system
and 166–7
summary 185
welfare model for working with
young offenders 170–71
young offenders 170–73
see also welfare of children
Society for the Prevention of Cruelty to
Animals 9
Society of Mental Welfare Officers
122
Solly, Henry 19
Specht, H. and Courtney, M.E. 54
Specht, H. and Vickery, A. 124–5
Speed, Maurice 136
Standing Conference of Organizations
of Social Workers 118
Starkey, P. 55
Stears, M. 45
Stedman Jones, Gareth 13, 33
Stein, M. 178–9
Stephens, T. 114
Stephenson, George 91
Stevenson, Olive 174
Stewart, Mary 31–2, 59, 61
Stouthard, Elmer 56, 64n1
Sturdy, H. and Parry-Jones, W. 66
suggested reading *see* further reading
Sukina 175
Sullivan, M. 152
summaries
Charity Organisation Society (COS)
34
commissioning, competences and
'social care' 161–2
'mental deficiency,' working with
82
radical voices, turbulent times
146–7
social work between the Wars 63–4
social work forerunners 17
social work high tide 125
social work with adults 203
social work with children and young
people 185
welfare of children 103
Survey 46
Szasz, Thomas 192

Taft, Jessie 56
Taylor, L., Lacey, R. and Bracken, D. 171
temperance movement 9, 21, 90, 99–100, 206
Thomas, J. 141
Thomas, Martin 133
Thomas, R. 213
Thomson, D. 68–9, 72, 79, 81
Tillyard, Frank 39–4141
The Times 128
Timms, N. 61
Titmuss, Richard 116, 209
Towle, C. 57
Townsend, D. 209
Townshend, E. 29
Toynbee, Arnold 22, 48n1
Toynbee Hall 36, 38, 39, 41, 45–6, 48n2
Training Organization for Personal Social Services (TOPSS) 157
Tredgold, Alfred 69, 70

Under the Cover of Kindness (Margolin, L.) 215
Union of the Physically Impaired Against Segregation (UPIAS) 152–3
Unitarian strand in reform movement 9, 11
United States 33, 45, 52–3, 56, 57, 61, 64, 67, 73, 124–5, 196, 215
   comparison with 54–5
Unofficial Secrets (Campbell, B.) 185n1
Utting, D., Rose, W. and Pugh, G. 183

Vice Society 9
Victoria, Queen 19
voluntary care committees 89, 101
   role of volunteers 89–90
voluntary organizations, activism of 9–10

Wagner Report (1988) 195
Waifs and Strays 90
Wakefield Board of Guardians 69
Walkowitz, D. 58, 211, 215
Waterhouse Report (2000) 180
Waters, Margaret 96
Waterson, J. 149
Webb, Beatrice 68
Webb, D. 146

Webb, John 147n1, 184, 197–8, 203n2
Webb, Margot 185n3, 197–8
Webb, Sidney 50–51, 68
Weinstein, J. 138
welfare of children 84–104
   adoption, change in legal framework and 96–8
   Adoption Act (1926) 98
   Adoption of Children (Regulation) Act (1939) 98
   adoption process, emergence of 97–8
   boarding out
      moves towards 87
      regulations concerning 87–8
   'boarding out' under the Poor Law 87–9
   child protection 92–6
   child rescue 90–92
   Children Act (1889) 93–4
   Children Act (1908) 95–6, 102
   children and Poor Law 85–90
   Children and Young Persons Act (1933) 102
   Church of England Temperance Society 99–100, 103, 206
   classification under Poor Law 85
   corporal punishment 85
   delinquency, social conception of 100–101
   exploitation 85
   families in 19th century 84–5
   family privacy, importance of 84–5
   fostering, moves towards 87
   further reading 104
   Guardianship Act (1925) 98
   'hooliganism' 99
   Howard League for Penal Reform 99–100
   juvenile crime, increase in 99
   juvenile offenders, work with 98–101
   local authority, legal framework change and role of 101–3
   local government supervision, calls for 88–9
   national probation service, establishment of 100
   National Society for the Prevention of Cruelty to Children (NSPCC) 92–6
   residential homes, development of 91

welfare of children (*Continued*)
   school attendance officers 101
   school care committees 89–90
   social work function with juvenile
     offenders, emergence of 99–100
   social work functions, emergence of
     88–90
   state involvement in, statutory
     development of 102
   statutory basis for adoption,
     pressures for 97
   summary 103
   voluntary adoption societies 97
   voluntary care committees 89, 101
     role of volunteers 89–90
   voluntary organisations and child
     rescue 90–92
   welfare organizations, emergence of
     90–91
   workhouse schools 85–6, 88
   workhouses, removal of children to
     86
welfare state 107–9
   key legislation of 109
   origins of 130
   social work within 133–6

Wells, H.G. 68
Welshman, J. 191
Westminster Hospital Gazette 59
Westwood, L. 80
Whelan, Robert 22, 33–4
White, Tom 107, 112, 113, 118,
   119–20, 120–21, 168
Willmott, P. 89, 90
Winnicott, Donald 108, 112
Woodroofe, K. 54–5, 212
Woods, Robert 38
Wootton, Barbara 114
Workhouse Visiting Society 36
workhouses
   removal of children to 86
   system of 35–6
   workhouse schools 85–6, 88

Yelloly, M. 55, 110, 112
Young, A.F. and Ashton, E.T. 12, 13,
   14, 42–3
young offenders 170–73
Younghusband, Eileen 110, 111,
   191
Younghusband Report (1959) 89, 111,
   115–16, 116–17, 206